Relief Beyond Belief

Exploring the World
of Natural Healing

Alexandra Barker

Ⓢ SERAPHINE PUBLISHING

Published by:

SERAPHINE PUBLISHING
29 Queen Street, Belleville, Ontario K8N 1T3
seraphin@reach.net   www.seraphinepublishing.com

National Library of Canada Cataloguing in Publication

Barker, Alexandra, 1958-
    Relief beyond belief: exploring the world of natural healing /
Alexandra Barker

Includes bibliographical references.
ISBN 0-9730187-2-0

1. Alternative medicine--Popular works. I. Title.

R733.B37 2002   615.5   C2002-904482-0

Printed in Canada.

Dedication

For probably as long as I've dreamed of writing a book, I've imagined its dedication. Now I discover there are so many people to thank, it's impossible to list them all; family, friends, the many wonderful therapists who shared their knowledge, and my visionary publisher. Still, there are those who deserve special recognition.

Relief Beyond Belief is dedicated to my mother in loving memory of my father, who guided me on this path; to my children, Richard, Reneé, Julieann and Justine, and especially to my sweetheart and soul mate Tony, who never let me give up.

Finally, I dedicate this book to you, my readers. I hope you enjoy reading *Relief Beyond Belief* as much as I have enjoyed creating it. May you always use it in good health.

Foreword

Back in Ontario just three weeks after a 20-year absence, I wanted to get one of my classes in natural healing going in the Brighton area. Little did I know Alexandra Barker and I were destined to meet.

I was on my way to the grocery store when I heard the phone ringing and ran back to answer it. Alexandra, a reporter, was looking for a story idea, and had time "right now" to interview me. She'd heard I had been teaching at the Natural Health Consultant Institute in Montreal and was looking to set up shop in my new home. Now, I know a knock on the door from the universe when I hear one, so groceries could wait, and Alexandra came over.

I hadn't been in town long enough to think about how to reintroduce my courses in spiritual healing, let alone figure out a class schedule or where to hold my workshops. Within the next hour or so, Alexandra had offered me her aerobic studio to hold a class, helped me choose a fresh title for a course, and assisted me in firming up dates for the class, which could then be published along with her story.

Alexandra has progressively been bursting onto the natural healing scene ever since, checking out complementary approaches to healthcare, immersing herself in everything from guided meditation to reiki training, and on to shamanic journeying, sound healing, feng shui and many other expressions of wellness. She continues to scour the county for healers, therapists, and other wellness practitioners, facilitators and teachers in her quest to nourish her own growth and that of her readers.

In *Relief Beyond Belief*, Alexandra has created a user-friendly guide to the world of complementary healthcare available in Northumberland County. She is the consummate journalist offering readers a collection of concise, detailed, practical and thoughtful descriptions of various natural healing modalities. This

book is a great resource for anyone interested in an unbiased intro-
duction to natural healing.

The value of *Relief Beyond Belief* really came home to me one
evening, when a physician friend of mine picked it up, opened the
book at random and began reading the chapter on Therapeutic
Touch. Here was the most doubtful set of eyes reading a rather
foreign approach to healthcare from an allopathic standpoint;
Alexandra's open and thoughtful description intrigued him.

Relief Beyond Belief is a wonderful resource in the world of
natural healing, and it is available right here in our own backyard.
I know Alexandra has tried and been positively affected by every
treatment she writes about. She has been so excited about these
transformative effects she wrote this book to share them with
everyone! I am honoured to be able to introduce this book, and all
of the valuable, healing resources it offers, to you. Use it in good
health.

Cheryl Storey, M.A.
Natural Health Consultant, Reiki Master.
The Angels' Attic: Training in Self-Healing.
Cobourg, Ontario.
June, 2002.

Table of Contents

Introduction

Dear Readers:

What an amazing time it has been, exploring all these natural healing modalities in order to present them to you!

My journey began a year and a half ago when the sudden death of a loved one sent me spiralling into despair, with virtually no sense of spirituality to sustain me in my hour of need. Yet as I witnessed his final struggle, and saw how strong his spirit remained despite his body's failings, I realized that we are truly more than just our minds and bodies. And in the midst of the darkness, a light began to glimmer.

In subsequent months a series of "coincidences" brought me in contact with many spiritual teachers and holistic therapists who generously shared their time, insights and knowledge with me. I became fascinated and set out to absorb all I could, immersing myself in workshops, reading voraciously, and putting into practice all that I had learned. The transformation was evident almost immediately; suddenly I had less need for aspirin and antacids, my old stand-bys for combating the effects of stress, and minor ailments I had accepted as my lot in life simply disappeared.

I was overjoyed to have these amazing new tools to draw on, and initially, that was enough for me. Soon, however, I began to realize how many people aren't aware of the many options available to them. A burning desire began to grow inside of me, a yearning to share my discoveries. This took the form of writing a series of feature articles on natural healing, which birthed the concept of *Relief Beyond Belief,* my literary equivalent of shouting from the rooftops!

What Your Body is Trying to Tell You

I realized while doing my research and learning more and more about natural therapies, that we have within our grasp the ability to improve our own health and well-being, naturally, by simply listening to the clues our bodies are sending us every day and responding to them. While you are reading this book, think of the signals your own body has been sending out. Try to listen to your own inner knowing. Your body will tell you where you have blocked energy. For example, headaches are thought to indicate two conflicting internal feelings, and can be eliminated by allowing both to have a voice; speaking your truth. Catching a cold indicates your body needs a rest, and an opportunity to get back into balance. Complexion problems indicate you are holding back your male energy (whether you are male or female) and need to take action or to express yourself more clearly. If a skin rash erupts, it indicates you are itching to do something. Ask yourself what, and follow your intuition.

Allergies indicate a lack of trust in your intuition and repressed feelings, such as sorrow or anger, and can be eased by expressing those feelings. If your allergy symptoms include watery eyes, it indicates you are suppressing sorrow. Back pain stems from the feeling that you have to support others, and the need to express your feelings. Lower back pain often indicates suppressed sorrow, while upper back pain often represents suppressed anger. Experiencing menstrual cramps indicates you haven't been listening to your inner female and need some quiet time to turn your attention within. Though some of the therapies and ideas in this book may initially strike you as totally bizarre (as they did me), they are, in fact, amazingly effective. This is but a select offering of complementary therapies; there are many more to be experienced as you start Exploring the World of Natural Healing!

How to Use this Book

Everything you think, every action you take, has an impact on your body. Our beliefs and thought processes play a huge role in what happens in our lives, directly influencing our health, even determining whether or not we achieve our goals. Whether you're dealing with nuisance ailments or facing a much bigger health challenge, *Relief Beyond Belief* will introduce you to the many non-invasive, drug free options that are available to you.

Relief Beyond Belief is your personal guide to natural healing therapies for the mind, body and spirit. It will give you a deeper understanding and working knowledge of the many complementary therapies available to help you achieve peak physical, mental and emotional health.

A common thread weaving these therapies together is the belief that the body is self-healing, and that symptoms should not be masked, but regarded as a message from the body that something is not right. If they're ignored, the body will send increasingly stronger messages until it gets our attention. And since each part of the body is interconnected, a disturbance in one area can cause problems in another, so it makes sense to get to the source of the problem and heal it. Several of these therapies also have the power to put you on the path of self-discovery. They have been arranged alphabetically in individual chapter form for easy reference. Enjoy in good health!

Please note, this exploration of complementary therapies is not intended to serve as medical advice. If you are pregnant, or suffer from cancer, high blood pressure, heart disease or other serious illness, consult your physician before attempting any of the modalities described in this book. They are not intended to replace conventional medical health care, though they work well with it.

Please also note that I am not medically trained or qualified and that any therapies described in this book are for educational purposes. Your choice to use any of the treatments found in this book and any results of that usage is your own responsibility. Complementary therapies should never be used instead of medical treatment. You should never stop taking or reduce any medication without first consulting your doctor.

For your convenience, and to help you on your path to natural health, a glossary of commonly used terms can be found in Appendix B. Also, at the back of the book, a directory of holistic practitioners in the Quinte and Northumberland Regions is included.

It's important for you to feel completely at ease with your therapist, so it is worthwhile to spend a bit of time talking with any therapist you are considering before committing to ongoing treatments. Avoid any who display self-serving characteristics. Your therapist should radiate health and well-being. If he or she appears tired or sick, it's possible that the therapist isn't able to harness life force energy adequately enough personally, let alone for others, and may drain your vital energy instead of boosting it.

Holistic health requires patience. Herring's Law, the universally accepted guideline for healing through homeopathic therapies, says to allow at least three months for improvement, as well as a month for each year the condition has existed. I encourage you not to let this dissuade you and to persevere. The results will be worth it.

If there is one concept I would most like to share with you, it is this:

What we are today
Comes from our thoughts of yesterday,
And our present thoughts
Build our life of tomorrow.
Our life is the creation of our mind.
— Buddha

Chapter One

Feeling Pressured?
Try Acupressure!

The thing always happens that you believe in,
and the belief in a thing makes it happen.
– Frank Lloyd Wright.

Pressure is something most of us try to avoid, but with this therapy, a little pressure in the right place is a good thing! It's very likely you've already used acupressure without realizing it — massaging your temples to relieve a headache is a classic example of using acupressure points to help the body heal. Acupressure can be easily learned and performed in the comfort of your own home, and is beneficial for any age group. Once you learn where your acupoints are located, you'll literally have a first-aid kit at your fingertips with which to self-treat headaches, cramps, and a wide range of other ailments.

What it Is

Acupressure, an ancient Chinese therapy, has been used to promote good health and to relieve pain, stress, and stress-related health problems for 25 centuries. Its healing properties are attributed to its ability to balance the chi flowing through the body's meridians. Meridians are invisible, interconnected energy channels located throughout the body. Stress, poor nutrition, and lack of exercise can disrupt the flow of chi, creating blockages that can eventually lead to disease. Applying pressure to specific acupoints along the meridians breaks up the blockages, allowing the chi to flow and the body to heal itself.

There are over 360 acupoints on the body. They are located all over the body, close to the surface of the skin in small hollows, usually between bones. Each acupoint has a specific effect on particular organs or body systems.

What it Does

Modern science explains acupressure by suggesting that it triggers neurochemicals in the body, directing the brain to relieve pain, reduce inflammation, and even to regulate appetite. Acupressure has been proven to relieve nausea and dizziness, and many practitioners report having good results using it to treat headaches, cramps, allergies, asthma, and carpal tunnel syndrome, along with stomach, liver, kidney, lung and heart problems.

A Typical Session

Prior to your first professional acupressure treatment, your therapist will obtain your medical background and details about your diet and lifestyle, along with information pertaining to the problem at hand. After taking your pulse the therapist will ask you to lie on a therapy table while he or she performs acupressure by firmly pressing or massaging the acupressure points to stimulate them.

Treatments take approximately one hour. No oils or equipment are used. Some points may feel tender, and you may experience discomfort or coolness, but this generally passes quickly. The number of treatments required depends on the ailment, and may vary from weekly visits to seeing the therapist as needed. See your doctor if ailments persist, and if pregnant, consult your doctor prior to having a treatment.

Try it Yourself

Though a trained practitioner will provide the highest level of help, you can learn to apply acupressure techniques on yourself or loved ones with a little practice. Acupressure points are slightly more sensitive than their surrounding areas, and can easily be found by probing gently with your thumb. Once you locate the point, hold

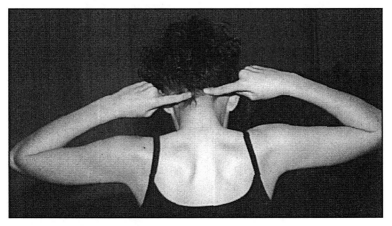

Julieann Gendron demonstrates the acupoints at the base of your skull. Pressing these points will relieve tension headaches.

your middle fingers at a 90-degree angle to the skin, pressing gently at first and increasing pressure to the point where you feel a mild sensation, which should not be painful. Tenderness generally indicates a lack of balance in the area.

Either hold a steady pressure or apply and release intermittently. Each acupressure point should be held for 10 to 30 seconds, up to two minutes. For best results, acupressure treatments should be done regularly, daily if possible.

Ready to give acupressure a try? First, a few words of caution. Don't apply pressure directly over genitals, arteries, scars, infections, ulcers or burns. A light touch is recommended when treating the stomach, as well as sensitive areas on the throat, below the ear, or the outer breast near the armpits. To avoid nausea, treatments should be delayed for an hour after eating. Fingernails

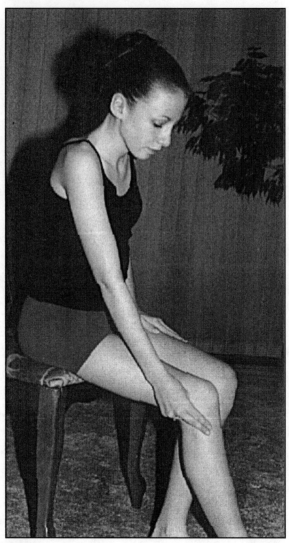

Apply pressure to your acupoints using the tips of two fingers.

should always be clean and smooth. It's also important to be relaxed and comfortable, and to maintain deep, relaxed breathing. Apply acupressure on the exhalation except in cases of swelling or extreme pain, when it should be applied as you inhale. Acupressure is even more effective when combined with visualization. As you apply pressure, visualize the condition improving and the part of the body healthy and functioning well. See Chapter 28, "Visualization" for tips.

Remedies for Common Symptoms

A daily facial acupressure treatment is a quick and easy way to help prevent headaches and sinus problems, and to improve the tone of your facial skin. Begin by placing each index finger beside the tear ducts, pressing against the bridge of your nose for 10 seconds. Then slide your fingers down the sides of the nose to your nostrils, and press and hold for 10 seconds. Next, press two fingers of each hand between your eyebrows and hold for 10 seconds. Then draw your fingers out to your temples, and press and hold another 10 seconds. This completes the cycle, which should be repeated three times a day.

Headaches can be treated by pressing the Third Eye acupressure point, found at the bridge of your nose between your eyebrows, for 15 to 30 seconds. This will help balance the pituitary gland and will relieve hay fever, indigestion, ulcer pain and eyestrain. Another headache remedy is to press the index finger of your left hand to your left temple, and the index finger of your right hand to your right temple. Hold for 15 to 30 seconds.

Insomnia and arthritis, headaches and neck pain can be eased by pressing your index fingers against your hairline, your left index finger one-half inch to the left of your spine, and your right index finger one-half inch to the right of your spine. Hold for 15 to 30 seconds.

To treat a toothache, press the Jaw Chariot acupoint, found at the end of jaw by the ear, on the side of face that hurts, and hold for 15 to 30 seconds.

Bronchitis, sore throats, chest congestion, heartburn and hiccups can be treated by pressing the acupressure point called

Heaven Rushing Out, located at the hollow of the base of your throat, and holding for 15 to 30 seconds.

Coughing and congestion can be relieved by pressing the acupressure points below your collarbone next to your breastbone and holding for 15 to 30 seconds.

Anxiety, cold sweats and insomnia can be treated by applying acupressure to the Spirit Gate point located outside the wrist, below the first crease in line with your pinkie, and holding for 15 to 30 seconds.

Suppress out of control coughing by pressing the point at the bottom of your biceps, slightly to the outside of your arm and holding for 15 to 30 seconds.

To treat tennis elbow, press the outside of the knuckle on the pinkie side of your opposite hand for 15 to 30 seconds.

Lower back pain can be eased by pressing two points located two inches from either side of your spine and holding for 15 to 30 seconds.

Disk and hip pain can be eased by using your index and middle fingers of each hand and pressing either side of your tailbone at the top of the crease in your buttocks for 15 to 30 seconds. This can relieve back and hip pain, or pain from a slipped or herniated disk.

To ease menstrual pain, use your index and middle fingers to press the Sea of Energy acupoint, located two finger-widths below the belly button. Hold for 15 to 30 seconds. This relieves PMS, menstrual cramps, and irregular vaginal discharge, as well as helping to correct irregular periods and constipation. Another technique to alleviate cramps is to press your index and middle fingers to the outside of your knee, three finger-widths below your kneecap.

To reduce hamstring pain, press the point midway between the back of the knee and the bottom of your buttocks on the leg that doesn't hurt. Hold for 15 to 30 seconds.

Knee, leg and lower back pain can be eased by pressing both thumbs to the Supporting Mountain acupressure point in the centre of the base of your calf and holding for 15 to 30 seconds.

Chapter Two

Aromatherapy is
Heaven Scent

*Smell is a potent wizard that transports us
across thousands of miles and all the years we
have lived. — Helen Keller*

Have you ever caught a whiff of perfume on a breeze and suddenly been transported to another time or place? Aromas have the power to evoke distant memories of people and places because out of all our senses, the sense of smell is the most strongly linked to the subconscious.

Scents are capable of producing immediate, intense responses because they are processed by the part of the brain that controls memory and emotion. The sense of smell is also strongly linked to many of our most basic survival instincts, such as our appetite and sleep functions. Aromatherapy is the practice of using this connection to create a sense of well-being and to promote healing.

Aromatherapy offers a gentle, soothing, and effective treatment for many conditions, including depression, anxiety, viral infections, malfunctioning organs and skin disorders, as well as improving circulation and memory. Aromatherapists use essential oils (pure, concentrated plant extracts) for their fragrance and ability to produce profound changes in the mind and body. They're particularly effective in treating stress-related conditions, and are frequently used as home remedies.

History

The practice of using essential oils dates back to ancient Egypt, Greece and Rome, when the extracts of specific plants' flowers, buds, roots, and bark were used to treat disease. It was revived in the 1930s when chemist Rene-Maurice Gattefosse burned his hand and plunged it into a container of pure lavender oil for relief. His hand healed within hours, leading Gattefosse and other scientists to pursue further experimentation and to develop aromatherapy treatments still in use today.

What it Does

Essential oils have varying physical and psychological benefits. Their properties can be antiseptic, warming, cooling, astringent, stimulating, soothing, relaxing, sedative, decongestant or antispasmodic. The highly concentrated, inflammable oils are extracted either through steam distillation or by cold-pressing a specific part of the plant. They're then mixed with a carrier oil such as soy or almond oil, or diluted in alcohol before being inhaled, applied to the skin or sprayed into the air.

Aromatherapists believe that certain aromas can improve your sense of well-being and can alleviate emotional disorders. Various studies that have measured the heart rate, muscle tension and skin temperature of test subjects before and after inhaling different scents support this belief. Studies demonstrate how aromas affect an individual's stress, behaviour and performance levels, establishing that inhaling certain fragrances causes a person's positive moods to increase, and negative moods to decrease.

Inhaled aromatic molecules stimulate odour-sensing nerves as they enter the nasal cavity, sending impulses to the limbic system that trigger a calming or energizing effect on the body, depending on the oil used. When combined with massage, they're absorbed into the blood and circulated throughout the body. Whether aromas work by stimulating glands to produce hormones that fight pain and inflammation, or by reacting with hormones and enzymes in the bloodstream, aromatherapy is currently enjoying the sweet smell of success as its popularity soars.

How to Use Them

Essential oils are available in liquid, semi-solid or solid forms, and can be added to massage oil, used in hot or cold compresses, added to a bath, or dabbed on pulse points.

Remedies for Common Symptoms

There are several ways aromatherapy can be used to bring quick relief in the home.

Aching muscles or strains can be soothed by massaging stimulating or relaxing oils into the skin. Use a prepared oil, or add about five drops of essential oil to four ounces of a carrying oil to create your own unique blend. You can also make a hot or cold compress by adding five to 10 drops of oil to four ounces of water. Soak a washcloth in the solution and apply to the area. Lie down and relax.

Suffering from sinusitis and other respiratory problems? Find quick, temporary relief by adding six to 12 drops of eucalyptus oil to a bowl of steaming water, covering your head with a towel, and breathing in the vapours. Keep a tissue handy, and eyes closed during this treatment.

For a soothing or energizing bath, try adding eight drops of essential oil to a full tub, or four drops to a foot or hand bath. Prefer showers? Simply soak a washcloth in the oil solution and apply to the skin while under the spray, though people with skin allergies should not use this form of treatment.

Spraying essential oil compounds in the air adds a pleasant fragrance to the room and promotes a sense of well-being and calmness for everyone in it.

Your Complementary Medicine Cabinet

Here is a list of some essential oils you may want to keep on hand, and the healing properties attributed to them:

Bergamot: Has a fresh, lively, citrus scent and an uplifting, encouraging emotional effect.

Cedarwood: Has a soft, warm, woody scent and a calming, comforting effect. It acts as a sedative, astringent and antiseptic. It is used to treat acne, oily skin, and dandruff. It promotes spirituality and balance.

Chamomile: Smells light and floral; is soothing and relaxing. Reduces swelling and treats allergic symptoms and digestive problems. Relieves stress, insomnia and depression.

Eucalyptus: Smells refreshing, clean and penetrating, and has a stimulating, cleansing effect. Lowers a fever, clears sinuses, relieves coughs, and has antibacterial and antiviral properties. Also used to treat boils and pimples.

Everlasting: Heals scars, and reduces swelling after injuries. Relieves sunburn, and fights bronchial and flu infections. Treats spasmodic coughs, whooping cough, shingles and herpes. It is also an anticoagulant, anti-inflammatory and a stimulant.

Frankincense: Has a spicy, woody scent and a calming, strengthening effect. Also acts as an antiseptic, an expectorant and an astringent. Used to treat nervous tension and anxiety, infections of the urinary tract, and hemorrhages. This scent is also useful in meditation as it slows and deepens the breath.

Geranium: has a clean, sweet, floral scent and a calming, balancing effect.

Juniper: Has a refreshing, fruity scent and an uplifting, detoxifying effect. It is also an antiseptic, astringent and diuretic. It is used to treat diabetes, cystitis and arthritis. It is thought to be beneficial in providing protection from negativity and danger when combined with visualization.

Lavender: Has a fresh, clean, floral scent and a soothing, relaxing and balancing effect. Heals cuts and burns, kills bacteria, relieves depression, inflammation, spasms, headaches, respiratory allergies, muscle aches, nausea and menstrual cramps. Also treats bug bites and lowers blood pressure.

Lemon Verbena: Has a clean, fresh, citrus scent and a stimulating, refreshing effect. Acts as a sedative and a purifier. Used to treat fever, hangovers and nervous indigestion. It is also thought to promote spiritual love.

Lemongrass: Has a sweet, grassy scent and a refreshing, rejuvenating effect. It has antiviral, anti-fungal and sedative properties, and is thought to stimulate psychic awareness.

Orange: Has a lively, fresh, citrus scent and a cheering, relaxing effect. Used to treat anxiety and intestinal gas. It also has the effect of plumping up dry, wrinkled skin.

Peppermint: Has a strong, mint scent and an invigorating, stimulating effect. Alleviates digestive problems, cleans wounds, decongests chests, and relieves headaches, and muscle pain. Also good for motion sickness.

Rosemary: Has a clean, strong scent and an uplifting, rejuvenating effect. Relieves pain, increases circulation, decongests the chest, relieves indigestion, gas and liver problems, reduces swelling, fights infection, and helps to treat depression.

Sandalwood: Has a warm, woody scent and a relaxing, sensual effect.

Tarragon: Stimulates digestion, calms neural and digestive tracts, and relieves menstrual symptoms and stress. Also treats hiccups.

Tea Tree: Has a strong, fresh scent and a cleansing, stimulating effect. Fights bacterial, fungal and yeast infections, and is used to treat acne, burns, insect bites, bladder infections, and vaginitis.

Thyme: Has an intense, herbal scent and a stimulating, strengthening effect. Eases laryngitis and coughs, fights bladder and skin infections, relieves digestive problems and discomfort in joints.

Vetiver: Has an earthy, woody scent and a comforting, balancing effect. Acts as a sedative and is useful in treating insomnia.

Ylang-Ylang: Has a sweet, flowery scent and a sensual, arousing effect. Relieves anger and physical pain, and is useful in treating impotence, depression and insomnia.

Chapter Three

Bask in the Glow
of Your Aura

What you can do, or dream you can, begin it;
boldness has a genius, power and magic in it. –
Goethe

A ura means, "glow of light", and refers to the electromagnetic field that surrounds and permeates our bodies like a halo. It is believed that our auras hold a record of all our past experiences as well as our current state of health.

What it Is

Your energy field actually has seven overlapping auras, which have been classified into three main layers. The first layer, the etheric body, relates to bodily functions and physical sensations, and ranges in colour from light blue to grey. A person with a sensitive body will have a bluish colour, while a more robust body will lean toward grey. It radiates from 1/4 inch to two inches from the body, and is in constant motion.

The second layer, the emotional body, follows the outline of the physical body. It is associated with emotions, and appears as coloured clouds in constant motion. It extends from one to three inches from the body. It contains all the colours of the rainbow, ranging from clear to muddy depending on your feelings at the time. Highly energized colours such as love or anger are bright, and confused feelings appear dark and muddy.

The third layer, the mental body, is associated with thoughts and mental processes. It usually appears as yellow light radiating around the head and shoulders and surrounding the body, extending three to eight inches from the body.

The fourth layer, the astral body, is associated with the heart chakra and our love for our mates and humanity. It extends six to 12 inches from the body. It also contains a rainbow of colours, though each is tinted with a rosy hue.

The fifth layer, the etheric template, is associated with higher will. It is connected to the fifth chakra which relates to the power of the word, listening and taking responsibility for our actions. It is considered to be the template for the etheric layer, which in turn is the blueprint for the physical body. It extends one to two feet from the body.

The sixth layer, the celestial body, is connected with celestial love encompassing all life forms. It extends two to three feet from the body. Through this layer you can achieve spiritual ecstasy with meditation and other means. This layer appears to be a shimmering light radiating from the body like a glowing candle.

The seventh layer, the causal body, extends from 2½ to 3½ feet from the body. It is associated with the higher mind and the integration of our spiritual and physical attributes. It contains all the auric bodies.

What it Does

Our aura changes in intensity of colour, size, and shape depending on our mental and emotional states, and also reflects our individual gifts and potential. Animals, plants and rocks also have auras.

The colours in a person's aura also reflect any negativity that a person is holding. They can also be used to diagnose a person's health and spiritual well-being.

Auras can be photographed through Kirlian photography, which uses high frequency electrical currents instead of light, a process discovered by Semyon Kirlian in 1908.

Try it Yourself

You can see your own aura without any special equipment through this simple exercise:

In a dimly lit room, fully extend your arms with the backs of your hands facing you, fingers slightly splayed and fingertips touching. It is helpful to hold up your hands against a white background, which will enable you to see the colours more clearly. Let your eyes look beyond your fingertips so your vision is slightly unfocused. Keeping your eyes softly focused between your fingers and the space beyond, you will begin to notice white light surrounding your fingers. As you slowly separate your hands you will see thin vapours of white light connecting them. You may even detect a hint of colour.

This exercise may require several attempts, as we are not accustomed to focusing our vision in such a manner, but with persistence you will be able to see your own aura, and perhaps those of others as well.

Chapter Four

Bowen Technique

*Our doubts are traitors and make us lose the
good we oft might win, but fearing to attempt. –
Shakespeare*

The Bowen technique is a very relaxing form of bodywork.
It involves a series of gentle, rolling moves made on soft,
connective tissue at key points on the body. The gentle, yet
powerful moves send impulses to the brain, which processes and
returns the impulses, realigning the body. By adjusting the combination of these moves, the therapist can target a specific problem,
or address the body as a whole.

History

The Bowen muscle/nerve/connective tissue technique was developed in Australia by Tom Bowen, who had no formal healthcare
training, but became very interested in relieving pain after being
exposed to a great deal of suffering while serving in World War II.
He discovered that when certain moves were performed on the
body, specific effects were produced. He continued to work with
this process for over 30 years. Bowen therapy is now practised in
Australia, New Zealand, The United Kingdom, and Europe. It has
recently made its way to North America.

What it Is

Bowen therapy, often called physical homeopathy, is essentially designed to stimulate energy flow, and to release tension and blockages, which allows the body to rebalance and heal itself. It is safe for all ages.

Bowen brings lasting relief from pain and discomfort by working every internal organ system in the body as well as the muscles and bones. It treats a wide range of problems and injuries, and it is an effective treatment for sports injuries, joint and muscle pain, arthritis, carpal tunnel syndrome, and gastrointestinal disorders. It is also helpful for respiratory difficulties such as asthma, colds, hay fever and sinus conditions. Migraines, PMS, fibromyalgia, diverticulitis and more are all treatable with Bowen.

A Typical Session

When you go to receive a Bowen treatment you'll be asked to remove your outer clothing and to lay on a treatment table covered by a sheet. The therapist will ask you to breathe deeply to relax your body, and will probably deep breathe along with you. The therapist will deftly press into strategic spots on your buttocks, using a comfortable pressure, then will leave the room, allowing your body time to react to the adjustment. In a few minutes the therapist will return, stimulate certain points on your knees, then leave again. You can expect this pattern of the therapist pressing specific parts of your body, then leaving the room, to continue throughout the procedure. Midway through you will be asked to turn over to allow the therapist to continue the treatment on the front of your body. Adjustments will be made to the base of your skull and arms, with breaks between each body part as described above. The series of moves take about an hour, and can be performed on skin or through light clothing.

The combined movements were designed to improve circulation, lymphatic drainage and toxin elimination. Bowen practitioners are trained to use "tissue tension sense" which allows them to detect stress build-up in muscle groups. The therapist then releases this tension through the Bowen techniques. The pauses are equally important, as they give the body a chance to benefit from each move and to return to its natural balance.

When the treatment is complete you will be advised to lay quietly for a few minutes to get your bearings. Then the therapist will assist you to a seated position to ensure that your spine remains perfectly straight. When getting off of the table you will be instructed to land with both feet on the floor at the same time, and to walk around the room several times to help with the integration process. You'll be asked to walk every 30 minutes throughout the rest of the treatment day to assist this integration. When arising from a seated position you should stand with your weight evenly distributed to help maintain the treatment's balancing effect. That night, while you sleep, Bowen's therapeutic effects will continue to work.

Ironically, the therapy may cause any pain being treated to briefly intensify before being relieved. Old injuries may also resurface before they are released. The process can be aided by drinking plenty of water, about three litres a day, and by taking relaxing walks. Hot baths, hot or cold packs and any other form of therapeutic bodywork, such as massage, chiropractic or acupuncture, should be avoided for five days after a Bowen session, as they may interfere with the treatment's effectiveness. Homeopathic medicine, essential oils and flower remedies are permissible.

Chapter Five

Every Breath You Take

*It is only when we forget all our learning that
we begin to know. – Henry David Thoreau*

One of the quickest, most efficient stress defence mechanisms is also the simplest available. No special equipment is required, you can use it anywhere, anytime!

To instantly calm yourself when you feel pressured by a stressful situation, simply stop and take a deep breath in. Exhale slowly and fully, consciously releasing any tension, feeling it flow out of your body and into the ground beneath you. Notice how your racing heart begins to slow as you take control over your response to the situation, and how quickly the negative physical effects of stress begin to dissipate.

We're all born knowing how to maximize the air we breathe to our body's best advantage. If you watch babies breathing, you'll notice their tummies rise and fall rhythmically, flooding their bodies with nurturing oxygen. As years go by, however, daily stresses cause the majority of people to abandon "belly breathing" for shallow "chest breathing", which uses only the tops of the lungs.

What it Does

Stress causes the diaphragm to partially contract, which reduces the amount of chest space the lungs can expand into, allowing less air to be delivered to the lungs per breath. To compensate for this we automatically take more frequent shallow breaths, triggering physiological changes that constrict blood vessels, causing further stress.

The brain is the first organ to suffer from the resulting under-supply of oxygen, making you even more susceptible to the physical effects of stress, a contributing factor in fatigue, depression, and anxiety. Shallow breathing can contribute to a wide range of stress-related disorders including migraines, high blood pressure and panic attacks.

In contrast, the practice of deep breathing reaps many benefits. Advocates of breathing therapy believe proper breathing helps psychological problems as well as physical ones such as PMS, asthma and insomnia. By inhaling fully, you supply your body with an abundance of oxygen, which is essential to every cell in your body. Deep exhalations help rid the body of pollutants and stale air. Deep breathing helps all cells, tissues and organs perform at peak levels. It also helps connect the body to the solar plexus, a veritable storehouse of potential energy. The key is breathing from the diaphragm, drawing air into the lowest and largest part of the lungs.

Try it Yourself

To fully understand the process of proper breathing, it helps to break it down into three stages. Sit with one hand on your abdomen and the other on your rib cage. As you inhale slowly, feel your abdomen expand as your diaphragm moves toward the abdomen, drawing air to the lower lung. Notice how the rib cage expands as your intercostal muscles pull air into the centre of your lungs, then into your upper chest. As you exhale slowly, feel how the air first leaves your lower lungs, then the middle, and finally the top of your lungs.

To gain a sense of the difference deep breathing can make, lie down and fully relax your entire body. Starting at your feet and slowly working up to your head, tense each body part for five seconds, then relax the muscle for five seconds. Once you are completely relaxed, place a book on your stomach. As you draw air deeply into the lower lungs through your nose, use your abdominal muscles to push your stomach out. Pull it in as you exhale, keeping inhales and exhales an equal duration. Practising this technique for 15 minutes twice daily will encourage automatic deep breathing.

Can't sleep? To stimulate the sleep reflex, sit up in bed and take a long, deep exhalation. Then, breathing through your nose, gently tip your head up slightly as you inhale, letting it lower again as you exhale.

Practising breath control can help you achieve many things. For example, in yoga, breathing techniques can be used as tools to strengthen the mind's control over the body. See Chapter 29, "Yoga", for more about breathing exercises.

The following yoga breathing technique called *Kapalabhatir* cleanses the respiratory system by eliminating large amounts of carbon dioxide and other impurities, and increasing oxygen intake. Contract your abdominal muscles quickly. This forces air out of your lungs and causes your diaphragm to rise. Allow your stomach to relax. Repeating this technique 20 to 50 times quickly for three to five rounds will enrich your blood and body tissues and will massage your stomach, liver and pancreas.

In alternate nostril breathing, known in yoga as *Anuloma Viloma*, your exhalation is twice as long as your inhalation, which strengthens the respiratory system and expels stale air and waste products from your entire body. It also calms and balances your mind. To perform this exercise, bend your middle and index fingers into the palm of your right hand; hold your thumb, pinkie, and ring finger extended.

1. Close your right nostril with your thumb. Exhale through the left, then inhale for four counts.
2. Close the left nostril as well and hold your breath for 16 counts.
3. Release the right nostril and exhale for eight counts.
4. Holding the left nostril closed, inhale through the right for a count of four.
5. Close both nostrils and hold your breath for 16 counts.
6. Release your left nostril and exhale for eight counts.

This completes one round. Repeat nine times for a total of 10 rounds daily.

Chapter Six

Contemplate Your Navel
with Chi Nei Tsang

The physician should know the invisible as
well as the visible man. — Paracelsus

Y ou may be surprised to learn that navels are like
snowflakes: no two are alike. Check yours out. Is it round,
or does it pull to the left or the right? Its unique shape
reveals your individual areas of tension and blockages to a Chi Nei
Tsang therapist.

History

Chi Nei Tsang literally means, "working the energy of the internal
organs". It is a non-invasive form of abdominal massage that uses
chi, breath, and massage to release stored emotion and tension, to
tone the organs, and to integrate the body, mind and spirit. The
ancient technique originated in China, where it was developed by
monks to help them detoxify, strengthen and purify their bodies in
order to achieve the level of endurance necessary to perform their
spiritual practices. It was virtually lost to the world before being
rediscovered by Mantak Chia, who studied the techniques and
brought them to North America in the last decade.

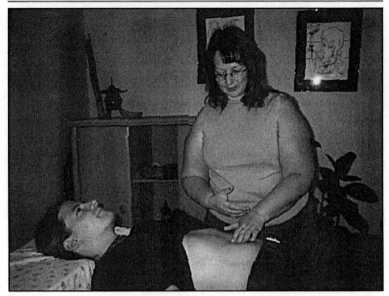

*Kim Bright Wallace performs a relaxing
Chi Nei Tsang treatment on Richard Leduc.*

What it Is

Chi Nei Tsang addresses the source of a person's health problems
and strengthens the body's immune system by massaging internal
organs as well as the digestive, respiratory, lymph, nervous,
endocrine, urinary, and reproductive systems. By massaging particular points in your abdomen a Chi Nei Tsang therapist can eliminate abdominal pain, detoxify and strengthen weak organs, aid
digestion, and release physiological and emotional blocks.
Beginning at the navel and working outwards, the therapist uses
deep, soft, gentle manipulation to train internal organs to work
more efficiently. Our "guts" actually contain more neurons than
our brains, and are the source of our feeling centres. This means
proper digestion and the elimination of toxins, including emotional ones, are necessary for peak physical, emotional and spiritual
health.

Chi Nei Tsang practitioners use the principles of Kung Fu and
Chi-Kung to stimulate neurons in the various organs and get to the
root of your health problems. They believe your body chi is trans-
formed throughout the body, becoming fire chi in the heart merid-

ian, water chi in the kidney meridian, wood chi in the liver meridian, metal chi in the lung meridian, and earth chi in the spleen-pan-
creas meridian. Different organs have specific properties associated with these five elements. Wood is associated with the liver, gallbladder and nerves as well as with frustration and excessive thinking. Fire is associated with the heart and small intestine as well as
with joy and anger. Water is associated with the kidney and bladder as well as with fear and creativity. Earth is associated with the
spleen, pancreas, and muscles as well as with worry and hate, and
metal is associated with the large intestine, as well as with depression and sensitivity.

What it Does

Chi Nei Tsang techniques initiate healing from within in several
ways. Their detoxifying effects rid the body of excess stagnation,
improving elimination and stimulating the lymphatic and circulatory systems. They restructure and strengthen by adjusting the
position of internal organs, releasing deep-seated tensions and
restoring vitality. The techniques balance emotions and help deal
with unprocessed emotions, one of the primary reasons for poor
health. The treatments include teaching self-help Chi Nei Tsang
abdominal massage techniques, enabling you to be more respon-
sible for your own health.

A Typical Session

Before beginning a treatment, which typically lasts about one and
a half hours, the therapist will conduct a preliminary interview to
determine the nature of your difficulties. During this interview he
or she will take notice of many things, including your tone of voice
and the presence of any nervous mannerisms, while watching your
eyes, ears, and face for any indication of imbalances.

Treatments are conducted on a massage or treatment table.
You will be fully clothed, but your abdomen will be exposed
enough to allow the therapist access to it. You'll be asked to take
slow deep breaths so the therapist can observe where you're holding tension. The therapist does this by watching your breathing patterns and noting which areas move, and which don't. The therapist

will generally breathe with you to help you keep your rhythm. This deep breathing promotes relaxation and enables the therapist to bring in more energy.

The therapist will begin a light massage, feeling where your internal organs are situated and how they feel on a physical level. Then the therapist will begin to sense how things feel on an energetic level. He or she will focus on the navel area first, taking note of its shape and which way its pulling, because if it pulls one way, organs in the opposite direction will be imbalanced as well. Using a slight pressure, your muscles and fascia (the connective tissue holding all the organs together) will be stimulated to help the organs shift back to where they should be and to encourage the navel to become more round. A gentle "cat pawing" of your abdominal region will stimulate your lymphatic system and will promote detoxification. Initially the therapist will massage very lightly, working within your comfort zone. Continually working with the breath, the therapist will gradually begin to work deeper, as you exhale. If the therapist discovers tightness he or she will continue to work in that spot, encouraging you to feel it also and to expand into the area with your breath while energy is directed there.

Treatments generally require four to five sessions. During that time, the therapist will instruct you on ways to continue the work at home to maintain the effects. Chi Nei Tsang is useful in treating chronic pain in the back, neck and shoulders as well as problems in the feet, legs and pelvis. On a personal note, I'd recommend you wait at least an hour after eating before having this treatment!

Chi Nei Tsang therapists practice qi gong exercises regularly to keep their energy up, and regularly teach their clients specific qi gong routines as well. See Chapter 22, "Qi Gong" for more information on exercises.

Chapter Seven

Colour Your World:
Colour Therapy and Chakras

The eyes of my eyes are opened.
– e.e. Cummings

What colour are you today? Are you feeling blue, or in the pink? A little green with envy perhaps? The fact that colour is such an integral part of our language reflects the powerful impact it has on us.

The colours we surround ourselves with affect and reflect our health and emotions, as well the image we project to others. Our eyes can distinguish approximately 1,000 distinct colours and thousands of shades and tints; we respond to them instinctively, feeling drawn to the ones that make us feel good.

History

Civilizations as early as the ancient Egyptians realized that colour had powerful energies, and used them as healing agents to help restore physical, mental and spiritual well-being. Modern science has established that our bodies need a daily minimum of 15 minutes of exposure to full-spectrum light (white light or sunlight) to maintain health and to prevent symptoms similar to jet lag.

What it Is

Colour rays are made up of varying light and energy frequencies, and each band has a different healing quality. Red, at one end of the spectrum, has a long wave length, a slow vibration, and a stimulating effect whereas violet, at the other end, has a short wave length, vibrates quickly, and has a calming effect. All colours have both positive and negative aspects; too much or too little can cause imbalance in our systems.

A Typical Session

Some colour therapists will use clairvoyance to examine your aura. Your aura is the electromagnetic field that surrounds your body and holds a complete record of your individual experiences as well as your state of health. The intensity of an aura's colours, size, and shape will shift depending on your mental and emotional state. See Chapter 3, "Auras", for more information.

Once the initial examination is complete the therapist will make a diagnosis and will suggest different ways of treating any colour deficiencies. Colours can be applied to the body physically, through exposure to light rays, or mentally, through visualization or meditation. The therapist may recommend that you simply eat more of a certain colour of food, change a decorating scheme to incorporate a specific shade, or add certain colours to your wardrobe. He or she may also balance your colours through meditation and creative visualization, leading you on an imaginary journey full of colour to balance the energy centres aligned with the spinal chord, called your chakras.

Once you become familiar with the energies associated with different colours you can let your intuition be your guide. A quick wardrobe check will reveal a preference for a particular colour; preferences or strong aversions to a shade is a sign that your body needs that particular wave length.

What Different Colours Represent

The colour waves we draw to ourselves radiate out to everyone we come in contact with, enabling us to have a positive impact on the world simply by harmonizing our colours. Each colour in the spectrum represents an emotional state, and can be used to treat different conditions:

Red represents passion and energy, and is a strong stimulant. Very little is used in colour healing because it can cause inflammation and over-excitability, though small amounts can be helpful in treating anaemia and depression.

Orange has a freeing action on the body, and is frequently used in colour healing because of the energy and the wisdom it imparts. Orange is also useful in promoting self-confidence, and healing nervous complaints.

Yellow, the colour of joy and happiness, has a cleansing and purifying effect on the body. It also stimulates sluggish digestion and enhances concentration.

Green combines the wisdom of yellow with the truth of blue. It acts as a harmonizer. It is beneficial for nervous complaints, and imparts peace of mind and clear memory.

Blue is soothing and promotes healing. It reduces fevers and blood pressure. It also acts as an antiseptic and a pain killer. It encourages the acceptance of things that cannot be changed, and brings calmness.

Indigo is a purifying colour that calms the mind. It is used to enhance psychic development, and is helpful in treating migraines and other painful conditions.

Violet helps treat all nervous and mental disturbances and is beneficial for lung disorders.

Chakras

A *chakra* is a central spot of energy located along the spinal column of the body. There are seven main chakras, each associated with a colour of the spectrum. Colour is closely associated with the seven primary chakras that correspond to the seven primary glands of the endocrine system. Each chakra pertains to a specific aspect of behaviour and development, and each vibrates at different frequencies. The three lower chakras, associated with basic emotions and needs, vibrate at a low level. They are associated with masculine or "yang" energy. The three higher chakras correspond to mental and spiritual functions, and vibrate at a higher frequency. They are associated with feminine or "yin" energy. The heart chakra, the fourth chakra located in the centre of the chakra alignment, is neutral, a combination of both masculine and feminine energies.

Though the chakras are harmonized in normal conditions, energy excesses or blockages can result in physical, mental and emotional imbalances. The blockages can be cleared, through colour therapy and other means, enabling the energy to flow undisturbed once again.

The root or base chakra, located in coccyx area in men and between the ovaries in women, is considered to be the root of physical vitality and basic survival urges. It regulates the suprarenal glands, kidneys, bladder and the spine. The colour associated with this chakra is red.

The sacral or sexual chakra, located just beneath the navel in front of the sacrum, is the centre of the ego and sexual energy. Other people's emotions are perceived with this chakra, which is associated with the gonads, organs of reproduction, and the legs. The colour associated with it is orange.

The solar plexus chakra is located just above the navel in the centre of the body, where physical energy is distributed. It is the centre of unrefined emotions, and is associated with the pancreas, stomach, liver and gall bladder. The colour associated with it is yellow.

The heart chakra, located in the middle of the chest, heart height, is the centre of unconditional affection, spiritual growth, compassion and love. It is associated with the thymus gland as well as the heart, liver, lungs and circulatory system. The colour associated with it is green, or pink.

The throat chakra is the chakra of communication, self-expression and creativity. It is associated with the thyroid gland, throat, upper lungs, arms and digestive tract. It is associated with the colour blue.

The third eye chakra, located in the middle of the forehead, just above the eyebrows, is the centre of extrasensory perception such as clairvoyance and telepathy. It is the seat of will, intellect, spirit and visualization, and is associated with the pituitary gland, the spine, the lower brain, the left eye, the nose and the ears. The colour associated with it is indigo.

The crown or lotus chakra, located at the top of the head at the fontanel, represents the highest level of consciousness attainable. It is the seat of intuition and direct spiritual vision, and corresponds with the upper brain and the right eye. It is associated with the colour violet.

Chapter Eight

Get Your Head Examined: Craniosacral Therapy

The most divine art is that of healing. And if the healing art is most divine, it must occupy itself with the soul as well as the body, for no creature can be sound so long as the higher part of it is suffering. – Pythagoras

When all else fails, you may want to consider getting your head examined. Craniosacral therapy, a procedure involving the gentle manipulation of the skull bones, has been particularly beneficial to people with chronic symptoms that haven't been helped by other forms of treatment.

History

The therapy was developed in the 1970s by osteopathic physician John E. Upledger with research compiled by Dr. William Sutherland, the father of cranial osteopathy. It operates on the premise that cranial bones are not completely fused, but are slightly flexible to allow for movement. Just as chiropractic has demonstrated that muscles can pull vertebrae out of alignment, cran-

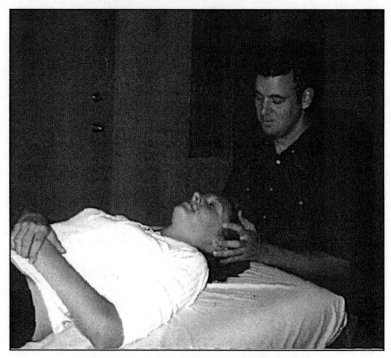

*A relaxing session: Michael Bruinix performs
craniosacral therapy on Justine Gendron.*

iosacral therapists believe taut muscles in the head can cause skull bones to shift on a microscopic level; enough to cause problems in the head and other parts of the body.

If one bone is inhibiting the movement of another on a microscopic level, it causes compression, resulting in headaches and other disorders. A nerve often has to wind and twist to go through little holes in the bones, so if the bone with the hole is also twisted, it impinges on the nerve. The goal of a craniosacral practitioner is to get the bone back where it belongs, allowing for clear conduction of the impulse, which clears up the problem.

What it Is

The premise of this therapy is that disorders such as headaches, sinusitis, and asthma can be caused by obstructions in the flow of cerebrospinal fluid in the brain and spinal cord. Therapists strive to remove these blockages by shifting bones in the client's skull, allowing the fluid to flow freely again.

The craniosacral system maintains the environment of the central nervous system. It is made up of membranes and cerebrospinal fluid that surround and protect the brain and spinal cord, and it extends from the bones of the skull, face and mouth to the tailbone. Any imbalances or dysfunction of this system can cause a person to suffer sensory, motor and/or neurological disabilities.

Though it is very subtle, the craniosacral rhythm affects every part of the body. Therapists are taught to monitor the rhythm at specific points to determine the source of any obstructions. These obstructions can be caused by repetitive strain injuries, blows to the head, illness, chronic tension, and other physical or emotional stresses or traumas. Using an extremely light touch they will then strive to correct any blockages in cranial rhythmic impulses throughout the client's body.

A Typical Session

During the treatment you can expect to remain fully clothed, though you may want to remove your shoes for comfort. You will lie on a treatment table, possibly covered by a blanket. The practitioner will support your head gently in his or her hands and feel for any imbalances in the flow of cerebrospinal fluid. The therapist uses his or her hands to "listen" for any irregularity in the fluid's rhythm. The underlying principle is that as soon as an imbalance starts, pain does as well, so wherever the therapist finds an imbalance he or she will subtly readjust the bones, and then will move on to the next area.

You may experience different sensations in your body during the 90-minute treatment, or you may hardly be aware of the therapist's actions, as sessions are as individual as the therapists and clients themselves. Throughout treatments therapists perform a procedure called Somato-Emotional Release, which promotes the release of tension in the body. This may prompt the client to remember past traumas or injuries. Re-experiencing and releasing these events helps the body reverse dysfunction and restore prior mobility.

Chapter Nine

To Sleep,
Perchance to Dream

A dream which is not interpreted is like a let-ter which is not read. — The Talmud

What did you dream about last night? Were you naked in public, did you make love to a famous actor, or were you in a play and forgot your lines? Or does the fantastic adventure you were just living usually vapourize like morning mist when you open your eyes?

Whether you remember them or not, scientific research shows everyone dreams about five times each night, and each dream can provide an entertaining glimpse into your psyche. Brain scans taken of dreaming subjects reveal that dreams are formed by drawing on emotional memories. Dreams occurring early in sleep tend to be about present situations, while morning dreams may recall aspects of the dreamer's early childhood.

We dream roughly two to three hours a night, as much as one-third of the time we're asleep. During this time our eyes follow dream sequences like a movie playing on a screen, known as rapid eye movements (REM), and our voluntary muscles remain para-lyzed for the duration. Being deprived of REM sleep not only increases the stresses of daily life, it leaves people feeling anxious and disoriented, and in chronic situations, can even lead to illness.

History

Some researchers feel a form of learning can occur during dream states, as in the cases of Einstein and Robert Lewis Stevenson, whose dreams led to significant breakthroughs in science and literature. Sigmund Freud theorized that dreams are the creation of unconscious desires such as sexual urges, and developed the free association method of dream analysis. In contrast, Carl Jung was more concerned with dreams' purpose than their cause, believing that they tapped into the collective unconscious.

The belief that dreams can promote healing can be traced back to the ancient Egyptians, who erected a temple to Imhotep, the god of healing. Ancient societies throughout the world believed that dreams could foretell the future, give guidance and facilitate healing. They felt dreams depicted actual soul travel, and that the waking world and dreaming world were really two versions of the same reality.

Dream Cycles

There are four phases to our sleep cycles. During the first phase brainwaves slow from the waking beta frequency to alpha frequency, where your muscles relax, your pulse, blood pressure and body temperature drop, and images begin to form in your mind. In the next phase, when we have most of our dreams, brainwaves slow to theta, and rapid eye movements (REM) occur. During the next phase, brainwaves slow to delta frequency, inducing a deep, dreamless sleep. Phase four is even deeper, with slower delta waves, resulting in a "dead sleep". These four phases are repeated approximately every 90 minutes, four or five times a night.

Dreams reflect what is happening in your body and mind, revealing truths about strengths and weaknesses that can be powerful tools in resolving emotional difficulties, unleashing potential, and improving health. Troubleshooting dreams can help solve problems by replaying disturbing events to help you arrive at constructive solutions. They can illustrate how lifestyle choices may be stressing your body or mind, as well as presenting a safe environment in which to experiment with new ideas, relationships, sex, and fresh approaches to situations.

Paying attention to your dreams can help you tap into inner wisdom, develop intuition, offer insights, assist spiritual growth. They can help you improve personal relationships, or forecast illnesses.

You can even set your intention of what you would like to dream. The tricky part is discerning your dream's real meaning, as dreams are often shrouded in mystery. This is because they originate from the part of the brain that developed before humans began communicating through speech. Instead of being literal interpretations, other people and animals are used as symbols to convey ideas, while lighting and colours reflect dream emotions.

Every dream serves a purpose and can teach you more about yourself. Even nightmares are not "bad" dreams. They often stem from traumatic events not fully experienced on a conscious level, and are your mind's attempt to resurface traumas so they can be released.

Keeping a dream diary beside your bed and writing your dreams in it as soon as you wake is an effective method for remembering your dreams. Note if a dream triggered thoughts of love or fear, and try to determine what it was trying to tell you. Describe it in the present tense, which allows you to stay more attached to its emotions and inner meanings, and include as many details as you can, as writing even a sentence or two will often trigger more of the dream to recall.

Many people find it helpful to hang a "dream catcher" near the bed where it will reinforce an intention to remember their dreams. Using a dream pillow filled with fragrant herbs such as lavender, rosemary, sage and mugwort to promote recollection and clarity may also help. It also helps to remove distractions such as televisions, radios and telephones from the bedroom, and to quiet the mind and body with meditation before going to sleep. A warm bath before bed promotes sleep, as does a before-bed snack of turkey, milk, bananas or cheese, all of which contain tryptophan, which has a sedating effect.

When it comes to dream interpretation, let your intuition be your guide. Begin with those you feel are your most important dreams, and try to ascertain their basic purpose. You may even give them titles to help determine their meaning. List key aspects, such as the setting and time of day, as well as elements like other people or animals that figure in the dream (seemingly external people and places actually depict your body, and mind, and your connection with others). Take note of any specific colours or numbers, as well as any actions taken and outcomes reached.

Dreams should be interpreted literally first, then symbolically. Dream dictionaries simplify this process, and have been used to determine the archetypal meanings of common dream symbols since the Beatty Papyrus was written in 1350 BC. However, if a particular definition doesn't ring true for you, simply discard it and delve deeper to discover what does. Remember, the symbols in your dreams evolved from your brain, and you are the best interpreter of them. Have fun exploring your inner world, and sweet dreams!

Chapter Ten

Energy Psychotherapy

When one door of happiness closes another opens, but often we look so long at the closed door that we do not see the one that has been opened for us. – Helen Keller

Is negativity ruling your life? Do you suffer from anxiety, depression and phobias? Do you have problems dealing with family issues? If so, you might want to consider consulting an energy psychotherapist to help you quickly resolve the issue.

Energy psychotherapy is a non-traditional form of psychotherapy. It is a non-invasive, gentle way of dealing with issues that can cause disturbances in your energy field. This therapy uses some traditional therapeutic tools, such as discussion and intuition, but also employs muscle testing to get to the root of the problem. In essence, energy psychology consists of defining what the problem is, deciding on a preferred state, and discovering what's stopping you from living the life you truly desire.

Perhaps your happiness is being blocked by a current life trauma, which could include prenatal and birth trauma. Or maybe a past life trauma is the culprit. Either way, once the block has been found and brought to consciousness, it can be removed by tapping acupressure points, by holding chakras, or by using affirmations or prayers.

What it Is

Energy psychology is based on the premise that any trauma we experience, be it physical or emotional, immediately imprints on our energy field, or aura. These traumas have a toxic effect, causing disruptions to our body's energy systems and compromising our life force.

Energy psychotherapy works with your complete energy field to change how you experience life, using muscle testing to determine what is preventing you from living the life you truly desire.

Energy psychotherapy approaches any illness on the premise that it has several possible causes: physical (such as bacteria, viruses, parasites, allergies, or toxic chemicals), emotional, or psychological. The objective is to treat all toxins related to the physical or emotional distress, so they will no longer support the disease. The psychologically and spiritually directed energy helps reduce, or eliminate anxiety, depression, phobias, hostility and other forms of negativity, removing these blocks to your happiness as you reprogram your energy field. Interventions or treatments can be as simple as tapping your own acupressure points.

A Typical Session

Therapists will typically ask you when the ailment started and what was happening in your life at that time in order to determine if there are any causal relationships between the two. They will compile a detailed life history to determine the nature of your school experiences, family relationships and any accidents or illnesses, to help them get to the source of the problem. Therapists endeavour to take away the effect of the trauma, so the incident can be recalled without the pain.

During treatments you will be asked to focus on the problem at hand while the therapist balances your chakras, which are believed to contain concentrated energy. They can become blocked with negative energy when there's been a trauma, which can be defined as anything that has a negative emotional or psychological affect on a person. By balancing the chakras the therapist eliminates the negative emotional charge associated with the situation, resolving the experience in a non-traumatic way and releasing it on an energetic level. Any negative emotions attached to it are removed, without altering the memory of the event or problem.

During therapy sessions you will be asked to hold your arm outstretched in front of the therapist, allowing him or her to muscle test while asking questions pertaining to your core beliefs. Then you repeat the question as the therapist attempts to lower your arm. If the sentence is true for you, the therapist will be unable to lower your arm; but if the sentence doesn't reflect your inner truth, your muscles will be too weak to resist the pressure.

Muscle testing, a form of applied kinesiology, bypasses what you think and taps into what a deeper part of you knows. The procedure is very useful for bringing unconscious beliefs to the foreground, where they can be resolved. Some consider it more reliable than a lie detector. Muscle testing enables the therapist to help you determine the real issues you're struggling with internally. Then the therapist can help eradicate roadblocks prohibiting your healing by clearing your chakras, removing trauma and relieving distress. Negative core beliefs can be eliminated, and replaced with positive core beliefs.

Energy psychology is reputed to successfully treat anxieties, low self-esteem, post-traumatic stress disorder, allergies, food sensitivities, and autoimmune disorders such as environmental illness. Many people report feeling immediate relief after a treatment. Energy psychology is compatible with many traditional forms of therapy.

Chapter Eleven

Flower Power

Bread feeds the body indeed, but flowers feed also the soul. — The Koran

Flowers are not only a delight to the senses, their essences can actually improve your health by getting to the emotional root that your problem stems from.

Flower extracts can treat a variety of unwanted emotional conditions by flushing out negative feelings, which many believe will also rectify any physical symptoms those emotions have created. Every plant and every flower remedy has its own signature vibration. When we ingest a plant's positive vibration, it helps shift our own vibration.

History

Dr. Edward Bach, an English homeopathic physician, developed flower remedies in the early 1900s. Bach believed that negative emotional or psychological states were the source of physical illnesses. He scoured the English countryside for flowers with healing properties, and experimented on himself to determine which flowers helped different emotional states. Through trial and error, he identified the 38 wildflowers used in Bach Flower Remedies, just one of the many branches of flower remedies now available.

What it Is

Bach was able to isolate a plant's vibration and to capture it in a medium of water, so it could be used internally to help shift negative feelings. Not interested in conducting studies proving his product to the world, Bach preferred to simply demonstrate how it worked and to allow people to prove it to themselves.

The flower extracts used are highly diluted solutions made from 38 different flowers called "mother tinctures". They are created by two means: the sun method, and the boiling method. In the sun method, flower heads are floated in a glass bowl filled with spring water in the sun for three hours. Then the flower heads are removed and the remaining energized water is mixed 50/50 with full strength 80 per cent-proof brandy. In the boiling method, flowering twigs are placed in a pan of spring water and boiled for half an hour. The pan is allowed to cool, then the plant matter is removed and the water is mixed 50/50 with 80 per cent-proof brandy.

Drops of the mixture are then further diluted in brandy and bottled for personal use. Patients are directed to put two drops in a one-ounce dropper bottle, fill it with mineral water, and refrigerate it.

Bach's intention was to create a simple, effective system that was easy to use, so people of all walks of life would be able to heal themselves. The remedies are used to relieve existing emotional difficulties, rather than to prevent them.

A Typical Session

Initially the therapist will choose remedies for you after talking with you, and helping you determine how you really feel and your personality type. Then you'll be able to choose remedies for yourself.

The flower extracts are also available in kits, a self-help system that doesn't require professional advice. Self-administered questionnaires help to select the correct flowers, which each correspond to a particular emotional or psychological state. It's recommended that no more than six remedies be combined at one time.

Following the treatment, you are instructed to pay attention to how you feel and the emotions you are experiencing.

Your Complementary Medicine Cabinet

Specific flower remedies can be used to treat a wide range of emotional problems. *Agrimony* is said to treat mental torture that hides behind a cheerful face. *Aspen* helps combat the fear of unknown things, while *Beech* helps the user increase tolerance levels.

If you have a hard time saying "no", *Centaury* is the essence for you, and if you don't trust your decisions, *Cerato* could help. *Cherry Plum* helps ease the fear of losing your mind, and *Chestnut Bud* helps those who fail to learn from their mistakes.

Chicory is the flower remedy of choice if you believe you are selfish and possessive with love, and *Clematis* could correct continual dreaming of the future without working toward those dreams in the present.

Crab Apple has a dual purpose, it is a cleansing remedy that also treats self-hatred. *Elm* helps those who feel overwhelmed with responsibility, while *Gentian* eases discouragement experienced after a setback.

If you feel hopelessness and despair, try taking some *Gorse.* *Heather* treats self-centeredness, and *Holly* addresses hatred, envy and jealousy. *Honeysuckle* is a good remedy for people who feel they are living in the past.

Hornbeam is a remedy for procrastination, and for individuals who feel tired at the very thought of doing something. Naturally enough, *Impatiens* is the recommended treatment for impatience.

Larch is the remedy to correct a lack of confidence, and *Mimulus* helps conquer fear of the unknown. *Mustard* is recommended for those experiencing deep gloom for no apparent reason. *Oak* helps people change the habit of continually pushing themselves past the point of exhaustion, and *Olive* helps ease exhaustion that follows mental or physical exertion.

Pine helps ease pangs of guilt, and *Red Chestnut* is the remedy for those who are overly concerned with the well-being of their loved ones. *Rock Rose* helps control feelings of terror and fright, and *Rock Water* helps to correct self-denial and self-repression.

If you feel unable to choose between two or more alternatives, consider trying the *Scleranthus* remedy. If you're experiencing shock, some *Star of Bethlehem* would be in order. *Sweet Chestnut* eases extreme feelings of mental anguish and hopelessness, and *Vervain* helps counteract over-enthusiasm.

Dominant and inflexible people would do well to take a dose of *Vine*, and *Walnut* helps ease concerns regarding change and unwanted influences. *Water Violet* helps to correct pride and aloofness, and *White Chestnut* is the remedy of choice to prevent unwanted thoughts and mental arguments.

White Oat is reputed to help clear uncertainties over one's direction in life, *Wild Rose* helps to off-set resignation and apathy. *Willow* eases self-pity and resentment.

There is also a pre-mixed remedy called *Rescue Remedy*, considered to be an emotional first-aid kit. It consists of five flower essences: *Cherry Plum, Rock Rose, Clematis, Impatiens*, and *Star of Bethlehem*. This blend is believed to immediately balance you and to provide relief and harmony during times of acute stress.

Users are encouraged to familiarize themselves with the remedies and to choose their own therapies. The recommended dosage is four drops of each remedy four times a day for as long as required. Flower remedies may be taken more frequently in times of crisis, with no risk of overdose or addiction.

Occasionally some emotions have been repressed for a significant amount of time, and must be cleansed from the body before they can be cleared. This can take the form of a rash, or a rush of unexpected feelings, and is not considered a reason to stop taking the remedy. When the emotional issue has been resolved, you may discontinue the treatment immediately. No weaning off is required.

Chapter Twelve

Harmonize with

Gemstone Crystal Therapy

Your diamonds are not in distant mountains
or in yonder seas; they are in your backyard,
if you but dig for them. — Russell Conwell

Crystals and gemstones are not only beautiful to behold, they can also have a profound physical and psychological impact on us. They're the simplest form of matter in the universe, representing every possible combination of energy, and for as long as people have walked the earth, civilizations on every continent have recognized them as being powerful tools for knowledge and healing.

Since crystals reflect the harmonies of matter and basic laws of nature, it's believed that bringing specific stones or crystals into your energy field can help correct any emotional or physical discord caused by an imbalance of these laws.

Every crystal consists of a single molecule repeated throughout its structure. This makes crystals fundamentally stable, maintaining a constant vibration and adjusting to environmental changes quickly. In contrast, your body is made up of thousands of different molecules, each with their own vibrational pattern and their own way of relating to their environment.

If you think of your bodily systems working together like an orchestra of individual instruments playing the same musical score, its easy to imagine how some instruments can go out of tune over a lifetime. When this occurs it becomes more difficult for other instruments to follow the score. A crystal's single vibration has the effect of a tuning fork on your internal orchestra, enabling your instruments to be re-tuned, thus re-establishing harmony.

What it Is

A crystal healing focuses on removing underlying stresses from your energy field. It can be combined with massage, reflexology, or spiritual healing.

A Typical Session

A typical crystal healing session would begin with the therapist obtaining a case history regarding your lifestyle and medical background. The therapist will choose specific stones for their healing properties and either place them around your body, or hold them during the treatment. Specific crystals can also be used to balance chakras. Gemstone/crystal therapy effects are believed to be cumulative, so practitioners may recommend monthly treatments for several months to maximize benefits. They might also suggest that you carry a specific stone with you, or that you take a gem essence, liquid versions of a gemstone's energy.

Try it Yourself

Colour plays an important role in crystal healing. Each colour has specific healing properties associated with it, because every colour has a physical, emotional and mental effect on people. A crystal's colour is dependent on how it interacts with light. Quartz, fluorite and corundum crystals come in many colours, and are given many names. For example, corundum is colourless when pure, known as a ruby when it's red, and as a sapphire when it's blue.

Your Complementary Medicine Cabinet

The following is a list of colours, the parts of the body they're associated with, and the crystals you can use to balance those areas:

Red is associated with heat, passion, and energy. It is the colour of the base chakra, which connects us to the earth and to our physical reality. It's associated with the feet, legs, hips, and the base of the spine. Some indications of red energy imbalances are difficulty with physical movement, circulation problems, hyperactivity, and exhaustion. A crystal healer treats these conditions with red stones such as ruby, jasper, garnet, granite and zircon.

Orange stimulates creativity on all levels. It's effective in healing, and is associated with the sacral chakra and the organs in the lower abdomen, the reproductive organs, and the kidneys. Imbalances are indicated by digestive disorders, lack of vitality, restricted feelings, and lack of focus. These would be treated with tiger's eye, amber, citrine, topaz, copper and carnelian.

Yellow, the colour of the sun, makes people feel happy and in harmony with their surroundings. It's associated with the solar plexus chakra and the upper abdomen and digestive system. Some examples of imbalances are nervous disorders, allergic reactions, arthritis, skin disorders, prejudices and lack of tolerance. A colour therapist would use stones such as yellow quartz, citrine and fluorite during treatments to relieve these symptoms.

Green is the colour of harmonious balance, growth and nature. It is associated with the heart chakra, the heart, lungs, diaphragm, arms and hands. Lack of discipline, abnormal growths, claustrophobia, lack of control, and invasive illness could indicate green energy imbalances, which might be treated with aventurine, jade, peridot, emerald, and dioptase.

Blue and indigo, the colours of flow and communication on all levels, are associated with the throat and brow chakras, and the neck, face, ears, eyes, nose, mouth and forehead. Laryngitis and tonsillitis indicate blue energy imbalances, as do congestion and creative blocks. Blue stones include celestite, sapphire, lapis lazuli, aquamarine, and azurite.

Violet combines the hot energy of red and the cooling qualities of blue, and is associated with the crown chakra, the skull, and functions of the brain, pituitary glands and pineal glands. Headaches, problems with the eyes and ears and the inability to concentrate indicate an imbalance of violet energy, which is treated with amethyst, fluorite, tanzanite, and iolite.

White, the vibration of pure potential, supplies whatever colour energy is needed. It is associated with the area above the crown chakra. White stones include opal, chalk and milky quartz.

Black contains all colours and absorbs all the energies into itself; it is a good grounding and protective colour. Black stones include jet, onyx, and obsidian.

Gem water and gem essences are liquid versions of a gemstone's individual energy. They can be used as simple, effective remedies, allowing the body to balance itself by dealing with underlying stress that is causing emotional or physical problems. Due to the atomic bonding between hydrogen and oxygen in water, water can hold the energy characteristics of the gemstone used. Its vibrations can then bring about positive changes. The advantage to using gem water and essences is that they allow the body to balance itself without causing unnecessary changes.

Gem water can be made by putting a clean crystal or gemstone in a glass pitcher filled with fresh water, and leaving it to stand 10 to 12 hours. One or two clear quartz crystals kept in a water pitcher will enhance water's beneficial effects.

Gem essences work on the same principle as flower remedies. Place a cleansed crystal in a plain glass bowl, cover the crystal with spring water, and let stand in sunlight for two hours. The water can then be transferred to a storage bottle containing 50 per cent brandy or vodka as a preservative to create a mother essence. Add three to seven drops of mother essence to a dropper bottle containing a 50/50 mix of water and brandy to create a stock bottle. A few drops can be added to bath water to energize the whole body and its aura, or the mixture can be sprayed into the air with a diffuser sprayer to change the energy of a room. It can be added to drinking water, or mixed with water to feed to animals and plants.

Be aware, caution should be exercised when considering gem water or essences as some minerals are toxic. Consult an expert or mineralogical book if in doubt.

Chapter Thirteen

Hypnotherapy

Go to your bosom; knock there, and ask your heart what it doth know. – Shakespeare

If your idea of a hypnosis is someone waving a gold watch before your eyes, intoning "you are getting sleepy", or convincing a group of people on a stage that they're actually on an amusement park ride, you're in for a pleasant surprise when you visit a certified hypnotherapist.

In my experience I was seated comfortably in the therapist's living room, with a spectacular panoramic view of Lake Ontario on one side and towering fir trees on the other. The hypnotherapist invited me to lean back, relax, and focus my gaze on a particular spot, her soft, melodic voice encouraging the stress of the day to simply melt away. Asking me to close my eyes, she mentally guided me down a hill and through a meadow to a sparkling stream, where I was invited to pass through a magical waterfall to another time, place, or even lifetime, with the intent of making life better in this one.

Hypnosis can be a useful tool to help you relieve stress, manifest goals, and kick negative habits. Some of the myriad benefits include pain management, alleviation of phobias and addictions, and enhancement of learning skills and creativity. It can be used to help reduce anxiety prior to an operation or medical procedure, as well as assisting in the post-operative healing process. Stress-related issues may be the most common reason people seek out hypnotherapy. Often they're unhappy, but don't understand the cause of their distress, which may stem from distorted core belief systems developed in their early years.

Negative self-talk, which sabotages self-esteem, often originates from an innocent remark. A parent or teacher telling a child "you're getting too big to wear that outfit," could be internalized by the child as "I'm too fat," leading to a preoccupation with weight throughout that person's life.

The therapist can help get to the root of a person's unhappiness and can help to resolve the issue. Hypnosis can be very effective in treating weight and smoking issues, sometimes in as few as one or two sessions.

Many people have preconceived ideas about hypnosis based on TV and stage shows, but the truth is that everyone drifts in and out of hypnotic states all day long. It's a natural state of being for people, as well as for many animals. When you daydream you're actually in the first level of a trance state, a light trance characterized by a relaxed body, slowed pulse and breath, withdrawal, and attention to an imagined activity or event. This is followed by a moderate trance, indicated by closed eyes, a loss of awareness of your surroundings, increased awareness of internal functions, more vivid imagery, and increasingly receptive senses. A deep trance would be marked by a further reduction of energy output, limp or stiff limbs, increased suggestibility, a narrowing of attention, heightened creativity, and a loss of awareness of your environment.

Once you are in a hypnotic state your subconscious will be receptive to suggestions such as "I am a non-smoker" or "I am more relaxed", which will then become beliefs that will modify your behaviour or produce a specific effect. There are six primary forms of suggestions: relaxation suggestions, deepening suggestions, direct suggestions, imagery suggestions, indirect suggestions, and posthypnotic suggestions.

As its name suggests, a relaxation suggestion has the effect of putting you at ease, inducing a state of receptivity and directing your focus inward.

Deepening suggestions take you to a deeper level of hypnotic trance, which the therapist may achieve by saying, for example, "you are so relaxed you're becoming one with the chair."

A direct suggestion may be a few words designed to trigger a certain response, instructing you to respond in a specific way, such as "when I count to three you will describe your first day of school."

An imagery suggestion will intensify other suggestions, setting the scene to try out new or reprogrammed behaviours.

There are two kinds of indirect suggestions. The first type would require you to focus on a desired emotional state by bringing to mind a memory that prompts this emotion, providing the therapist with a posthypnotic cue. With the second form, personalized metaphors are used to achieve specific goals. Posthypnotic suggestions are used to modify behaviour, such as increased confidence, or to eliminate habits, such as smoking.

It's very easy for most people to enter a hypnotic state, and while it is common to have concerns about losing control of the situation or saying something out of character, you're always in charge and cannot be made to say or do anything contrary to your values.

Most people seek hypnotherapy to relieve health problems, to increase self-esteem, to reduce stress, to improve athletic performance or to increase creativity. Many also use it to experience age regression or past life regression to examine events that may help them resolve current issues. Everything we experience is stored in our subconscious mind, which many believe also holds memories of past lives that can be triggered from events in this life.

When conducting age or past life regression the therapist will begin by easing you into a meditative state, helping you clear and focus your mind, then guiding you back into a memory from this lifetime or a past life. The memories won't necessarily be traumatic, and are often quite pleasant, though you may experience anger or sorrow as you relive past memories that may account for difficulties currently being experienced.

A Typical Session

Your initial visit with a hypnotherapist may last up to three hours while he or she establishes a rapport with you, gathers important information, and explains the basis of hypnosis. The hypnotist may show a few examples of the technique, and discuss whether this is the appropriate modality for the problem you've come to have treated. Subsequent sessions can range from one to three hours.

It's impossible to predict exactly how sessions may be required to treat a particular condition, as clients are as unique as their reasons for seeing a hypnotherapist. Hypnosis can be dangerous in certain conditions, which is why therapists only use hypnosis for pain management after a client has seen a doctor and has obtained a signed consent. A good therapist will not take on a client under a psychiatrist's or psychologist's treatment without the doctor's written consent.

Chapter Fourteen

The Eyes Have It:
Iridology

The eyes are the windows of the soul.
— Shakespeare

Eyes are often called, "the windows of the soul", but they can also provide a clear view of the physical body, from the inside out.

Your irises hold a medical history of your entire body. Iridology is the process of examining your iris to determine your state of health. It's been in existence since the earliest civilizations and is considered a form of reflexology, though it doesn't involve the practitioner actually touching the eye.

History

Modern knowledge of iridology dates back to 1670 when Phillipus Meyens charted the locations of body parts as they pertain to the iris. Over 200 years later, Dr. Ignatz von Peczeley, considered the father of iridology, caught an owl in the garden, accidentally breaking its leg. He noticed a mark that appeared in the owl's iris, and watched it slowly fade to a small dark imprint as the leg healed.

This prompted a lifelong study of the iris and its markings, and the publication of his eye chart in 1881.

What it Is

There are approximately 500,000 nerves connecting the eyes to the brain, continually relaying impulses to and from all parts of the body, giving the iris an up-to-the-minute account of its conditions. Imbalances in the body are often reflected in the iris long before there are clinical manifestations of disease.

The structural pattern your iris' fibres and colour variations gives iridologists a complete picture of your current state of health. They will assess the condition of your eye tissue to determine if any inflammation, congestion, toxic build-up, overactivity or underactivity exists. Though a practitioner is unable to name specific diseases, an analysis can interpret many things, including spinal misalignment, nutritional imbalance or endocrine imbalance.

Iridology is a good starting point for anyone on a quest for good health because it reveals inherent genetic strengths and weaknesses. A qualified iridologist will be able to tell you what conditions you came into the world with, as well as any illness or injuries that have occurred over the years.

What it Does

While iridology can't diagnose or cure a disease, it's a useful tool for looking at the structure of the body and for discovering its weaknesses and strengths. It can also monitor a person's return to health as dark areas of the eye lighten. Iridology is limited in some ways; if an operation has been performed under anaesthetic, for example, the iris will have no record of it, as nerve impulses will have been blocked. Interestingly, if an organ has been removed, the iris will retain the last recorded impulses from that organ.

Iridology can reveal if your body's primary nutritional needs are being met. It also can show the inherent strength or weakness of your organs, glands and tissues. It can also reveal your body's overall strength or weakness by revealing which organs are in most need of repair, or if there is any toxic settlement in the organs, glands or tissues. It can also determine if any inflammation exists in the body and what stage it is at, such as sluggishness of the bowel, circulatory problems, and much more.

Iridology cannot reveal the condition of your blood pressure, blood sugar levels, or specific laboratory test results, though it can reveal a lack or excess of a substance. It cannot determine specific drugs you may be taking, or surgical operations you've had. It cannot determine diseases by name, reveal if an operation is needed, or differentiate between drug side effects and the symptoms of diseases.

A Typical Session

During your initial consultation with an iridologist you'll be asked to complete a detailed questionnaire addressing any health concerns you may have. This helps the iridologist determine which part of your body needs work. The therapist will then take a picture of both of your eyes using a special camera. Once the photos have developed, the therapist overlays them with transparencies showing all the different systems of the body. The therapist then examines the photo of your irises and interprets their colour, shape and fibres, as well as any light and dark areas. This will reveal if any part of your body is struggling with disease or stress. Light areas of the eye indicate overactive areas; darker areas show underactivity. The iridologist will be able to pinpoint inherited strengths and weaknesses, and will be able to analyze the causes for any acquired imbalances. These results will be discussed with you during a follow-up appointment.

Rather than name a disease, the practitioner will describe an area as overactive or underactive. For example, the practitioner wouldn't be able to tell for certain if you have an ulcer, but might notice that the part of the iris representative of your stomach tissue is underactive. They will then be able to direct you toward optimum health by recommending corrective measures you can use with your diet and lifestyle.

While not a therapy in itself, iridology is a useful tool for analyzing the cause of someone's illness, as well as for monitoring a person's return to health.

Chapter Fifteen

Kinesiology

I think I can, I think I can, I think I can!
— Watty Piper

I think I can, I think I can, I think I can... or do I really? The children's story, *The Little Engine That Could,* by Watty Piper had a valuable lesson for us all. As the little train struggled up the side of a mountain it kept repeating to itself, "I think I can, I think I can." Of course, being a children's story, the little train succeeded, and the children's toys were delivered. But if the little train were human, chances are its subconscious would have countered with a chant of "I'm not so sure about that," making for a dramatically different ending.

What about you? Do you have underlying beliefs that conflict with what you consciously think, holding you back from what you want to accomplish in life, or perhaps even making you ill?

There's an easy way to find out. Manual muscle testing bypasses what you "think" and taps into what a deeper part of you "knows". The procedure is very useful for bringing unconscious beliefs to the foreground, where they can be resolved. Using muscle testing to communicate directly with the body is an integral part of applied kinesiology.

History

Applied kinesiology, meaning, "the study of body movement" was originated in 1964 by chiropractor George Goodheart, who established a relationship between muscle weakness and other physical, mental and emotional conditions. It operates on the premises that each muscle is connected to particular organs or body systems, and that if a muscle isn't working properly it will create problems in its related body part. Applied kinesiology is based on the belief that energy flows throughout our bodies, and if it is disrupted through illness or stress, our bodies will weaken.

What it Is

Applied kinesiology is renowned for being able to determine the underlying causes of health problems that can otherwise be hard to diagnose. It addresses emotional, nutritional and physical conditions, as opposed to simply looking at symptoms. Through muscle testing, the systems of the entire body can be balanced and restored to maximum functioning. This increases energy and vitality, prevents illness, improves posture, and relieves pain and tension. It's particularly beneficial for determining food allergies.

A Typical Session

Muscle testing consists of a therapist placing the client's arm or leg in a particular position, and isolating a muscle in order to gauge its response to gentle pressure. A muscle's normal response is to lock against resistance. If the muscle response is weak, it indicates low energy in the meridian system to which that muscle corresponds. As a weak muscle response to a verbal question indicates a negative answer, therapists can ask questions to assess a response to any stimulus. This enables them to locate and correct energy imbalances, and to restore health and well-being through a wide range of treatments.

A kinesiologist would begin a treatment by obtaining your medical history, and then would examine you to determine the cause of the problem, be it a lack of energy, a nutritional deficiency, or a physical disorder. He or she will use muscle testing to see if you can maintain an arm or leg position while slight pressure is applied to it. If you cannot maintain the position, the therapist will proceed further to find out why, and if there are any areas that require re-balancing.

Once the therapist has pinpointed the problem areas he or she will use a light touch to massage pressure points related to these areas. Stimulating these points increases the flow of blood and lymph fluid to the muscles. Following the treatment you may experience some tenderness for a day or two as the toxins dissipate, but you generally should feel an overall sense of well-being.

Applied kinesiology encompasses all aspects of an individual: mind, body and spirit. It is a valuable form of preventive medicine, and can help people change damaging belief systems and behaviours, and manage emotional issues better. It can also improve artistic skills, athletic performance, and even reading and writing skills.

Try it Yourself

There are several self-help methods for using applied kinesiology that can be particularly beneficial in handling emotional stress. Stimulating your emotional stress relief points (the small bumps located on your forehead midway between your eyebrows and your hairline) can help you cope with distressing situations. Holding these points draws the flow of blood to the front of the brain where objective decisions are made, and away from the back of the brain which relies on old memories and experiences. This removes the situation's emotional charge, enabling you to find new solutions.

To begin, sit or lie down in a comfortable position, closing your eyes and placing your fingertips on the bumps. Think about what's bothering you, focusing on it until the thoughts fade away. If you can feel pulses under your fingertips, wait until they synchronize, which is a sign the treatment is complete. Then open your eyes and think about the situation again, and notice if you feel any changes. If you find you're focusing on a different aspect of the same problem, clear it the same way.

By holding the emotional stress release points you can rewrite the past or create a positive outcome for a future event. Hold the points and imagine how you would like a scenario to play out, creating a favourable outcome. Visualize yourself being comfortable in the situation, and play the scenario over in your mind several times. This technique can be used to relieve any stressful situations, or to improve your performance in any situation.

There are other self-help applied kinesiology procedures you can use to further your personal development. If you've been unable to achieve a particular goal, there may be underlying factors at work leading you to unconsciously sabotage yourself. When your unconscious belief differs from that of your conscious mind (known as "psychological reversal") it can wreak havoc with your life, but there is a way to correct it. Locate the acupressure point on the outside of the hand, halfway between the base of the pinkie finger and the wrist. Using two or three fingers, tap on the point for 20 seconds while repeating out loud, "I profoundly and deeply accept myself and all my problems and shortcomings."

The temporal tap is another technique that can help you change unwanted habits and negative thought patterns, and can reinforce positive ones. Temporal tapping penetrates the sensory system filter, allowing new information into the nervous system. To use this simple, effective technique, make a positive statement such as "I have stopped smoking" while tapping the left ear from front to back, then a corresponding negative statement, such as "I no longer need to smoke" while tapping the right ear from front to back.

Brain Gym® is an extension of educational kinesiology developed by Dr. Paul Dennison to help children with learning difficulties. It has also proven to be beneficial for people of all ages, helping in a number of ways like preparing for academic tests, overcoming fear, changing habits, handling stress, developing creativity, training for sports, and enhancing social skills. Brain Gym® offers a simple, inexpensive approach to many challenges and usually produces results in a few sessions. The movements promote effective communication among the nerve cells in the brain and body, stimulating mental alertness, improving memory and increasing self-esteem.

Chapter Sixteen

Step into the Magic of Labyrinths

The trail is the thing, not the end of the trail.
Travel too fast and you'll miss all you are
travelling for. – Louis L'Amour

If you feel like you've been going around in circles in life, it may be time to seek out a labyrinth. You'll still be walking in circles, but at the same time you'll be tracing an ancient pattern of healing, with each step bringing you closer to resolving the puzzles of your life.

As you navigate a labyrinth's elaborate twists and turns, meandering your way toward your ultimate goal — the centre — you'll feel a sense of calmness descend over you. Perhaps this explains why labyrinths have been considered a universal symbol of healing and renewal of the body-mind-spirit connection for 3,000 years.

Labyrinths have long been used as meditation and prayer tools, and as models of life's path. The ancient symbol is a combination of a circle and a spiral, a metaphor representing the journey to our own centre and back out into the world.

Ancient and modern labyrinths can be found in most parts of the world. Perhaps the most famous of all is the Chârtres

Labyrinth, a medieval stone labyrinth found at Chârtres Cathedral, in France.

In the past decade labyrinths have become popular in North America as well. Made from many materials, they have been painted on canvas, constructed out of stone, brick, and sand, and even carved in turf grass.

Unlike a maze, a left-brain puzzle consisting of many paths, false leads and dead ends, a labyrinth is a right-brain tool using intuition, creativity and imagery to follow the one winding path leading into the circle and out again. Labyrinths can be used in several ways. They are used as walking meditations, or as exercises to gain an understanding of the human psychological and spiritual journey. Different images and metaphors can also be introduced to accentuate the experience.

A Typical Experience

There are three components to the labyrinth walking experience. The walk to the centre calms your thoughts, allowing you to be fully present in your body. Arriving at the centre connects you with your inner guidance, while the walk out leaves you empowered and ready to transform your life.

Before entering the labyrinth, walkers are advised to take a moment; relax, focus on the present moment, and release as much tension as possible. You may want to say a prayer or to focus on a question that you would like answered. Or you could simply ask yourself what you need in your life right now, being open to any answers that come to you as you walk the path.

Once inside a labyrinth, take your time and walk at your own pace. Be mindful of your life, envisioning your life's goal and thinking about what the turns represent to you. When you reach the centre, which can take 20 minutes or more, spend some time in contemplation. The journey back out invariably feels different than the one in, and it is beneficial to be aware of your different impressions.

When the labyrinth walk is completed, take the time to reflect on the experience. It is said that anything revealed within the labyrinth offers valuable lessons to the labyrinth walker, so pay attention to every detail of the experience.

Chapter Seventeen

Magnetic Field Therapy: Do You Have a Magnetic Personality?

There is a great difference between the power that removes the invisible causes of disease and that which merely causes external effects to disappear. – Paracelsus

History

The practice of using one of the strongest natural forces in the world to promote vitality dates back to Ancient Egypt, when Cleopatra enhanced her "magnetic personality" by adorning herself with magnetized lodestones. Paracelsus, one of medicine's most prominent physicians, also believed life force was influenced by magnets, and today an estimated 120 million people worldwide use magnetic field therapy for natural pain relief and to promote good circulation, energy and stamina.

What it Does

Magnetic field therapy affects people in several ways: by affecting change in calcium ions allowing them to heal broken bones faster or to direct calcium away from arthritic joints, by increasing or decreasing endocrine hormone production, and more. Magnets achieve these benefits by exerting a pull on charged particles in body fluids, increasing the flow of blood in the areas the magnets are placed on, and by increasing the level of oxygen and nutrients in the blood, relieving the toxicity causing the pain.

Years of research have established that magnetic fields stimulate every cell in the body, creating the ideal environment for the body to heal itself. When magnets are applied to the body, magnetic waves pass through the tissue, creating secondary currents that reduce pain and swelling.

Every magnet has a north and south pole. The north pole side is believed to have a calming effect, while the south pole side is thought to stimulate.

Magnets increase the body's potential to heal by promoting energy flow and lymphatic circulation in the area influenced by the magnet, helping the body cells to function at their optimum level. They are used to treat a wide variety of conditions, including carpal tunnel syndrome, menstrual cramps, sinus headaches, arthritis, fibromyalgia, osteoarthritis and more.

Magnetic field therapy is generally used as a short-term aid to promote recovery from injury, but may also be used regularly to promote health and vitality in treating chronic conditions. When used to treat injuries such as broken bones, cuts and burns, magnets have been shown to significantly reduce healing time and scarring. In some cases, magnet therapy has reduced and even reversed chronic conditions such as cancer, degenerative joint conditions and some forms of arthritis. However, they are not endorsed here as a cure for any disease or symptom. Always consult your doctor before beginning any new treatment.

Magnets are available in many forms: small discs, attractive jewellery such as bracelets, necklaces and earrings; pads and seat cushions for the car or home; mattress pads, and even hair brushes and shower systems. Shoe insoles reputedly enhance the body overall and drinking from a magnetized mug is thought to aid digestion and the absorption of nutrients.

Magnet therapy is also effective for animals. Pets suffering from arthritic pain may benefit from a magnetic pet pad, collar, or blanket.

Magnetic field therapy works differently for everyone. Experiment with different types of magnets and their placement. In some instances, you may feel the benefits of magnet therapy almost instantly, though in other cases it may take several weeks.

When choosing a magnet, it's important to remember they aren't all created equal; this is a case where the adage "you get what you pay for" is true. So think long-term investment, bearing in mind a good quality magnet will retain its power for the lifetime of the user. Many magnetic field therapists will use applied kinesiology to muscle test you with magnets to see if magnets increase your level of strength or not. See Chapter 15, "Kinesiology" for details.

Since magnets are effective for approximately 75 per cent of the population, many magnetic field therapists will lend you the product you intend to purchase to try it out first, to ensure it will work for you.

Though magnets don't necessarily remove the underlying causes of pain, which may return when the magnets are removed from your body, they can provide an effective, drug-free alternative for relieving symptoms. Magnets should not be used by pregnant women or by anyone using a cardiac pacemaker or defibrillator.

Chapter Eighteen

Massage Therapy: Ah, There's the Rub

*The physician must be experienced in many
things, but assuredly in rubbing, for rubbing can
bind a joint that is too loose, and loosen a joint
that is too rigid. – Hippocrates*

Lying comfortably in a softly lit room, soothing music playing in the background and aromatic fragrances wafting through the air while all the tension you've been holding is expertly stroked out of your body, you may wonder — can anything that feels this decadent really be good for you? The answer is a resounding yes! And the benefits of massage are definitely time-tested.

History

The medicinal properties of massage therapy have been recognized for centuries. In fact, massage is widely considered to be the original form of natural healing. Touch is one of the first senses to develop, and is essential to our well-being; without it, a person can be left feeling depressed and isolated. Through touch, the art of massage can treat specific health problems and can provide a blissful escape from the routine of daily life.

Our skin is actually considered one big sensory organ. An area the size of a quarter contains over three million cells, up to 340 sweat glands, 50 nerve endings, and three feet of blood vessels. It acts as our third lung and third kidney, storing nutrients, vitamins, minerals, chemicals and waste. Massage is one of the most pleasant and relaxing ways of giving your skin the stimulation it needs to make nutrients available to the body, and to move wastes to where they can be processed and eliminated.

Studies have shown massage is effective in reducing the heart rate, lowering blood pressure, increasing blood circulation and improving range of motion. It increases blood flow, stimulates nerves, stretches and loosens muscles, and provides relief from anxiety, insomnia, depression and muscle pain. It promotes healing and helps eliminate pain by increasing the blood supply to contracted tissue.

What it Is

There are many different forms of massage therapy that offer immediate and long-lasting benefits. They are also effective in managing and reducing pain.

Some traditional massages include neuromuscular massage, a technique in which concentrated finger pressure is applied to painful muscle areas or acupoints. Deep tissue massage uses slow strokes and deep finger pressure on areas of chronic muscle tension or soreness. Sports massage, used to assist training and to prevent or help heal injuries, is beneficial in the treatment of sprains, strains and tendonitis. Manual lymph drainage, a technique using rhythmic pumping to help move lymph fluid through lymph vessels, is an effective treatment in cases where lymph nodes have been removed, or if radiation has been administered near them.

Many massage therapists use the five basic Swedish massage strokes developed by Per Henrik Ling in the late 19th century. Effleurage (slow, rhythmic strokes following the direction of blood flow to the heart) is a technique frequently used at the beginning of a massage to warm and relax the muscles. The therapist will typically use his or her whole hand, gradually increasing the pressure applied. This may be varied by stroking with fingertips, knuckles, or the heel of the hand.

The friction stroke, a steady pressure or small circular motions across muscle fibres, is used in areas around joints. "Tapotement", or drumming on broad areas of the body such as the back, can include beating with the side of the fist, cupping (striking with fingertips and the heel of the hand), hacking (using rapid chopping with the edge of the hand), and clapping (striking fleshy parts of the body quickly with a flat hand). The petrissage stroke involves kneading, pressing and rolling muscles, and when using the vibration stroke the therapist spreads his or her hands firmly over your body and rapidly shakes an area.

Some massages that are lesser known in this part of the world include Lomi Lomi Hawaiian massage and Hot Stone Massage. Lomi Lomi is an ancient healing art that's been part of the Hawaiian culture since the start of its oral history, and is now being shared with the western world. Lomi Lomi elders believe their ancestors are present during each session, helping guide them in their efforts to *maloma ola na o lwi*, "preserve the health of the people". True to ancient tradition, modern practitioners will typically say a prayer to invoke the presence of the elders to help guide their hands toward healing.

Lomi Lomi can be either light or deep tissue work, and involves rubbing, stroking, kneading, pounding, vibrating, pulling and compressing performed in a loving and peaceful manner; it may involve the use of a Lomi Lomi stick. Made from a guava tree found in the rainforest, the smooth stick is oiled and used to provide a constant pressure on backs, legs and acupressure points.

The main difference between Lomi Lomi and other types of massage is that it's intentionally spiritual in its approach to healing, targeting your mind, body and spirit. Lomi Lomi is believed to treat both the body and spirit by bringing healing energy into the therapeutic session. Because it is believed to connect the bodies and souls of two people, it is said to create a bridge through which a natural flow of energy and communication can occur.

A hot stone massage is very effective in treating stiff, sore muscles and arthritis. In this therapy approximately 48 heated stones are used with oils to massage the entire body. The heat has a relaxing effect on your muscles, and the stones limit the therapist to a medium skin depth, ensuring a pleasant, relaxing massage. Hot stone massages are relatively new to the western world, but have been part of Lomi Lomi massage for centuries.

A Typical Session

A therapist will usually ask you to fill out a complete health history prior to your first treatment. This is followed by a short interview and assessment, allowing the practitioner to isolate any problems and to establish an effective plan for you based on your individual level of discomfort and areas of concern.

Treatments are generally conducted in a private room equipped with a massage table, low lighting and relaxing music. Though some treatments require you to remove most of your clothing, professionals treat privacy with utmost respect at all times. Aromatherapy oils are often used during treatments to heighten the sensory pleasure and health benefits of massage. Massage therapy is useful in treating injuries such as sprains, strains, tendonitis, bursitis, migraines, tension headaches, whiplash, and many more conditions. Though massage cannot cure serious medical conditions, it has been proven helpful with the care of premature infants, HIV infection, chronic fatigue syndrome, asthma and more, in addition to aiding general health and well-being: benefits that last well beyond the hour or two spent on the massage table!

Chapter Nineteen

Meditation Made Easy

*[God] cannot be found in noise and
restlessness. God is the friend of silence.
See how nature ... grows in silence; see the stars,
the moon and the sun, how they move in silence ...
we need silence to be able to touch souls.*
— Mother Teresa

Have you ever been so engrossed in an activity that time has simply flown by without you being aware of it passing? Then you've experienced a form of meditation. Meditation simply refers to a way to focus our minds, and to tap into our own inner stillness, increasing our vitality and well-being on all levels.

Meditation isn't just simply emptying your mind of all thoughts and letting it go blank. That's pretty much the equivalent of training your mind to be a rock: unthinking, unfeeling, and stationary. Meditation is the opposite: training your mind to focus deeply on a desired subject, to the exclusion of everything else.

Everyone wants to be happy and to avoid suffering, but few people understand how to go about achieving that. Most people continually seek happiness externally through jobs, partners and possessions, devoting nearly all their time and energy to acquiring things outside of themselves. But the truth is, none of these things bring lasting pleasure, because both happiness and suffering are states of mind. The only true, lasting source of happiness is internal peace, and meditation has the power to create a calm, peaceful mind, which generates this inner peace.

Left to their own devices, our minds are constantly in motion: churning, agitated, and out of control, like an excited puppy running around sniffing at everything. Conversely, a disciplined mind is a peaceful mind. Meditation harnesses the strength of the mind, making it more powerful and giving us mastery over it, essentially training that puppy to sit and stay.

What it Is

Meditation can be as simple as focusing on your breath. Transcendental meditation involves mentally repeating a mantra, and mindfulness meditation, based on the Buddhist tradition *vipassana*, focuses on the present moment. You begin by scanning your body from head to toe, focusing on any areas that have pain or disease. You might follow this by focusing your attention on every inhale and exhale. But whether you follow a traditional form of meditation (such as sitting before a candle) or an active meditation (like walking), training the mind through regular meditation will gradually lead you to a purer form of happiness and will help you respond to changes in your life more readily. Eventually you will be able to remain happy at all times, even in difficult circumstances. Practising meditation for 15 to 20 minutes a day will calm your mind, reduce stress, and make a lot of problems fade away.

What it Does

Meditation's effects on the electrical impulses flowing through the brain can be measured with an electroencephalograph (EEG), which shows that meditation boosts alpha waves, the brainwaves which occur when you are very relaxed and peaceful. It also increases synchronization of the left and right brain hemispheres, lowering stress hormones and improving circulation. Meditation is proven effective for reducing stress, tension, anxiety and panic, as well as reducing high blood pressure and chronic pain. Many people say it improves memory and reduces the desire to use alcohol or drugs. It has been shown to reduce cardiovascular disease, and to relieve mild depression, insomnia, irritable bowel syndrome and PMS.

Try it Yourself

The habit is more easily formed if you stick with a scheduled time, preferably in a place you enjoy where you will not be disturbed. It may be helpful to set up a shrine for objects that inspire you, such as pictures, candles or incense. The best times to meditate are when you first wake in the morning when your body is rested and relaxed, and before supper, as a big meal may induce sleepiness.

All you really need is a quiet place where you can meditate undisturbed, sitting comfortably or lying down, with some point of focus for your mind, like your breath, a candle, a religious symbol, or a mantra repeated rhythmically. A basic breathing meditation is a good place to begin.

Lie down or sit in a chair with your feet on the floor, holding your hands loosely in your lap. Your shoulders should be level and your back straight but relaxed. This will allow your energy to flow more freely, and you will be able to comfortably meditate for longer periods of time.

Your mouth and jaw should be relaxed with your teeth slightly apart and your tongue resting against the back of the upper teeth, which will prevent excessive salivation and dry mouth. Bend your head slightly forward so your gaze is on the floor in front of you. Your eyes can be closed, or slightly open to allow light in and to prevent you from falling asleep. Remain as still as possible, letting any random thoughts pass by like clouds drifting through a summer sky.

Take a few deep breaths, allowing your body to settle as you let go of busy thoughts and distractions. Bring your attention inward; simply become aware of yourself in the room. Then spend about two minutes becoming more aware of feelings and sensations in your body. Scan your body from head to toe, mentally releasing any tension. Bring your attention to your forehead and temples and allow tension to melt away. Then let your face and head completely relax. Now focus on relaxing your neck and shoulders, arms and hands. Become aware of your chest and breathe naturally. Relax your hips, legs and feet. Using the power of your mind, totally relax your entire body until you feel comfortable and centered.

Now, focus on the natural rise and fall of your breath. Focus on the sensation of air entering and leaving your body. You may find it helpful to count in cycles of 10 complete breaths, starting at one again whenever your mind wanders. Whenever you become distracted, release the images or feelings and focus again on your breath. Continue for 15 to 30 minutes. At the end of your meditation, notice how relaxed and peaceful you feel, then try to maintain that state of mind throughout your day.

It is very important not to bring expectations to your meditation, as the meditation experience will change from day to day. In the beginning your mind will be hard to restrain, like that new puppy, but perseverance will pay off before long. Regardless of your initial results, you should feel good, for making the effort to meditate is in itself a meditation, as well as an accomplishment.

Chapter Twenty

Nutritional Therapy:
We Are what We Eat

Let your food be your medicine,
and your medicine be your food. – Hippocrates

We really are what we eat. When you consider that every part of our bodies was once food, it makes good sense to pay attention to the tools we're giving our bodies to work with. Good nutrition can help combat anything from the common cold to chronic illness. But realizing that what we eat and drink plays a huge role in how well the body functions is one thing; providing the body with all the nutrients it needs is another. Sometimes our conscious and subconscious have very different ideas about what they want. It can be a challenging task, and nutritionists agree many of us are falling down on the job. The *Canada Food Guide* provides a good guideline, but many people don't eat as well as it advises. Busy lifestyles can be a significant factor, lending themselves to poor nutritional habits. Also, many foods are devitalized due to soil depletion, and don't contain the vitamins we think they do.

History

Nutritional therapy began in the late 19th century when naturopaths such as J.H. Kellogg, Vincent Priessnitz and Sebastian Kneipp combined nutrition and fasting to cleanse the body and to increase its ability to self-heal. It has since developed into a sophisticated health care system using physiology and body chemistry to achieve a therapeutic effect. This therapy explores where your health has gone wrong, and shows you how to correct it through nutrition and an understanding of how the body works.

What it Does

Our bodies show signs that can indicate nutritional imbalances long before they become chronic illness, like brittle nails and hair, or mood swings. Many problems respond readily to nutritional therapy, including migraines and headaches, irritable bowel syndrome, PMS, high cholesterol, sinusitis, and some forms of mental illness. It also plays a vital role in helping the body fight cancers, heart disease, diabetes, and multiple sclerosis.

Minerals are considered to be important nutrients, and are involved in biological processes that allow you to process fats, carbohydrates and proteins. There are over 20 essential nutritional minerals, including calcium, copper, iron, and zinc, that play an important part in our day-to-day biological functions. A lot of foods common in our North American diets, like pop for instance, not only provide no nutritional value, but actually strip our bodies of vital minerals, leaving our bodies depleted.

A Typical Session

A nutritionist will begin by conducting an in-depth lifestyle analysis to appraise your diet, your stress levels and your exercise habits. Then, the nutritionist will determine where to recommend changes. For example, your body may need a ginkgo supplement to aid circulation, or vitamin C to improve bone mass. Then the nutritionist will determine if you have any food allergies or sensitivities, if you have a toxic overload due to chemicals in the environment, if you have poor elimination of waste products, or any nutritional deficiencies due to poor diet or special needs. The nutritionist will develop a regime for you to follow to combat any depletions that are discovered.

Many of today's nutritionists focus on prevention, and some offer diagnostics such as hair mineral analysis to assess your nutritional mineral status and to gain an accurate view of what's been happening within you over the past year. Hair mineral analysis is a new diagnostic tool in clinical nutritional medicine and holistic medical treatment that determines any nutritional mineral deficiencies and heavy metal toxicities in the body. Essentially hair mineral analysis involves the client cutting a tablespoon-size sample of hair, which is sent to a lab for analysis. Then the therapist will determine how to improve the situation and balance your nutritional needs.

Your nutritionist will probably advise you to take small steps and to make changes gradually, rather than attempting radical overhauls. Even small changes can reap big improvements in stress and energy levels, and people tend to incorporate small changes into their lives much more easily. Moving too quickly can cause you to feel nauseated, emotionally distressed and exhausted. Take it slowly. Some simple steps include eating a variety of whole fresh foods, and avoiding fast foods, which are riddled with preservatives and create more waste for your body to eliminate. Prepared foods are generally high in salt, preservatives and chemical additives and should also be avoided whenever possible. You may also want to consider switching to skim milk, or to a non-dairy alternative, choosing low fat cheeses, and eating chicken or fish more often than pork or beef.

If there is any single thing people can do to improve their health, it's increasing their water intake. Sometimes called the "forgotten nutrient", water is vital to every cell; small wonder when you consider we are made up of 70 per cent water. Too little water can lead to kidney, liver and bowel problems, as well as a lack of energy and a problem complexion.

Clean, pure water is a gift to the body, and while the recommended eight to 10 glasses daily may be hard to adjust to initially, if you give it a try for a six weeks you'll notice a big difference. It takes a while for your body to realize that it doesn't need to store water; it's actually getting the amount it requires. You shouldn't rely on thirst as a guide; by the time you feel thirsty, you're already partially dehydrated. Try having a glass of water whenever you feel tired or sluggish or have difficulty concentrating. Clear, odour-free urine indicates you're drinking enough water. Drinking a sufficient amount not only flushes out toxins; it slows the aging process, diminishing wrinkles and moisturizing dry skin by hydrating from the inside out. It can also help you shed excess weight by keeping you feeling more full, however its best not to drink it with your meals, as it will slow your digestion.

Try it Yourself

When considering ways to increase the nutrient value of your food, don't overlook herbs — you may have nutritional power-houses in your garden or growing wild in the backyard, though pre-pared herbs may be easier to obtain and use. An herbalist will be able to determine if your body is out of balance, and will recom-mend herbal remedies to restore your vitality.

Herbs

Medicinal herbs are defined as any plant possessing parts used for medicinal purposes. They have been used since the dawn of time, and are categorized as nourishing, tonic, sedating or stimulating, and potentially toxic. Herbs are used in two ways: internally through teas, tinctures, syrups, capsules, nose sprays, enemas, eye-washes, eardrops and suppositories, or externally through baths, ointments, compresses, poultices, soaps, masks and body wraps.

Your Complementary Medicine Cabinet

The following plants and herbs can be used to correct a variety of conditions.

Black cohosh (cimicifuga racemosa): Gives hot flashes the cold shoulder, and is also used to treat PMS and menstrual problems. This is a potentially toxic herb. Ask a trained herbalist before using.

Chamomile (matricaria recutita): Relieves tension and soothes sore tummies.

Dandelions: Rather than spraying or pulling them out by the roots, why not try adding a few leaves to your salad? Young dandelion greens are packed with nutrients such as iron, potassium, calcium and vitamins A and C.

Evening Primrose Oil (oenothera biennis): Useful for fibrocystic breasts, eczema and arthritis.

Feverfew (chrysanthemum parthenium): Relieve migraines by chewing a few leaves.

Garlic: Eating 10 or more cloves of raw garlic daily will fight viral and bacterial infections.

Ginger: Good for treating nausea.

Hops (humulus lupulus): Can be used as a tea to induce relaxation and sleep.

Purple coneflower (echinacea purpurea): An antiviral immune system stimulator reputed to reduce the length and severity of flu and cold symptoms.

Stinging nettle (urtica dioica): Rich in vitamins and minerals, is a potent diuretic and can be used to treat hay fever.

Violets: Violet leaves are highly nutritious and can be eaten in a salad.

Nourishing herbs such as nettles and lemon balm are very nutritious and can be used every day for long periods of time. Tonic herbs such as dandelions, ginseng and hawthorn support particular organs or systems and have a cumulative, preventative effect. Poppies, passionflower and wild lettuce are sedating herbs, while ginger and primrose are stimulating. Rue, goldenseal and black cohosh are powerful, potentially toxic herbs. Long term use could lead to addiction. Expert guidance is highly recommended when using herb therapy. Please follow the advice of a trained herbalist.

You may want to ask your nutritionist about the bioidentical hormones and enzymes now available to treat the symptoms of menopause. Bioidentical hormones are extracted from plants or genetically engineered in a lab. They are very similar to the ones naturally occurring in the body, and are available in several forms.

Chapter Twenty One

Polarity

Learn to get in touch with the silence within yourself, and know that everything in life has a purpose. – Elizabeth Kubler-Ross

Polarity therapy is based on the belief that all life is energy in motion; energy which makes up every living thing and all matter, which comes from and returns to a source. It combines healing therapies from the East and West, using energy-based bodywork, diet, exercise and self-awareness to restore health.

History

Polarity therapy was originated by Dr. Randolph Stone, a chiropractor, naturopath and osteopath. He spent his 60-year medical career investigating energy work and the healing arts, looking for a unifying principle to explain all forms of healing work. He believed the human energy system, like a battery or magnet, has positive and negative poles through which energy flow. He concluded that life is movement, flowing from positive through neutral to negative and back again, and that all pain is blocked energy. He believed that the human energy field is affected by touch, diet, movement, sound, attitudes, relationships, life experience, trauma and the environment. Stone felt there was only one true disease:

the disturbance or blockage of the flow of life energy, and that all pain and illness was a manifestation of energy imbalance.

What it Is

Polarity therapy maintains that energy states (neutral, positive and negative), should be maintained between particular parts of the body and the five energy centres that relate to them. The five energy centres are: ether, earth, fire, water and air. Ether is said to control the ears and throat. Earth controls the rectum and bladder. Fire controls the stomach and bowels. Water controls the pelvis and glands, and air controls the circulation and breath.

Polarity works with the human energy field, which, it is believed, holds mental, emotional and physical experiences. It views health as a reflection of the energy field's condition. Good health requires that the complete energy field is balanced, with the life energy flowing smoothly, and no areas of excess or depletion. Polarity therapists strive to find and dissolve any blockages, allowing energy to flow normally and maintaining the energy field in an optimum way. They endeavour to create balance through energy bodywork, nutrition, and counselling, giving you several tools with which to create a balanced life. It complements and supports many other holistic health therapies.

What it Does

Polarity consists of energy bodywork designed to reduce tension in the body and to balance life energy. In addition to discovering where your body needs releasing on a physical level, practitioners try to find the underlying energy patterns, listening to your personal energy flow with their ears, eyes and hands. They use touch and manipulation to detect breaks in the flow of energy in your meridians, using three types of pressure: neutral pressure (using only the tips of the fingers), positive pressure (using manipulation over the whole body except the head), and negative pressure (using a firmer touch and deeper manipulation).

The exercise component involves various stretches, including sitting cross-legged on the floor, squatting, and sitting with your hands behind your back. The positions are said to open the channels that carry the body's energy, and to strengthen the muscles, ligaments, and the spine. You may be asked to yell while performing the exercises as a tension reliever.

Mental attitude is another component of polarity. This may involve counselling, encouraging people to have a positive outlook on their lives, which is essential for harmony within the body and mind. Negative attitudes are thought to increase a person's susceptibility to disease.

A Typical Session

During your first session you'll be asked to complete a case history. The therapist will then do an assessment of your energy, testing reflexes and using pressure point testing to see if there are any imbalances in your flow of energy. Then he or she strives to promote balance and restore your natural flow of energy through a combination of hands-on bodywork, exercise, and nutritional guidance. The therapist will encourage you to work though any negative feelings you may have, and will help you develop strategies to resolve stresses in your life.

A single session may include several different healing techniques, such as acupressure, craniosacral therapy, osteopathy, chiropractic, naturopathy, reflexology, massage and yoga. They are generally 60 to 90 minutes long. During this time the practitioner will support you with his or her own energy, using a light to deep touch on specific areas of the body to stimulate your own natural healing ability. As you become more aware of the subtle, healing energetic sensations, you may experience them as tingling or warmth, resulting in deep relaxation and a sense of relief from problematic situations.

Since life force cannot flow freely through a toxic body, a purifying diet of fresh fruit, vegetables and fruit juices is often recommended to rid the body of toxins caused by pollutants and unhealthy eating. This is usually recommended for a period of two weeks. After the cleansing diet is completed, it is replaced by a nutritional diet to increase health; then a maintenance diet is prescribed to allow the newly achieved level of health to continue.

Energy bodywork is used to evaluate and to move energy to dissipate blockages and to balance energy systems. Exercises such as gentle stretching and yoga are employed, as well as listening skills to uncover unconscious patterns.

Polarity therapy is beneficial in helping you become aware of the underlying sources of your discomfort, rather than specifically diagnosing or treating disease. By restoring the natural flow of energy, therapists will help increase your overall health and sense of well-being. Benefits may include profound relaxation, new insights into your energy patterns, a strengthened immune system, increased circulation, improved nutrition, and increased stamina, creativity and self-awareness. In addition, it provides you with the tools necessary to maintain balance and wellness.

This therapy doesn't address specific diseases, but focuses on your overall health instead. To be effective, polarity requires your total commitment to the prescribed diet, the exercise routine, and the rest of the program.

Chapter Twenty Two

Qi Gong

No one can give you wiser advice
than yourself. – Cicero

What it Is

Qi gong, pronounced "Chee-gong", is an ancient Chinese healing tradition dating back 2,000 years. This blend of meditation, movement and breathing is said to reap powerful healing benefits, similar to those of tai chi. Its gentle breathing and meditation exercises help circulate energy and get the body back into proper alignment. It has been credited with reducing stress and anxiety, lowering blood pressure, boosting the immune system, and slowing aging. It also increases brain levels of serotonin and endorphins, producing a calming effect. Qi gong practitioners use the exercises to treat migraines, diabetes, prostate trouble, impotence and pain, as well as to improve fitness and general health.

What it Does

Qi gong stimulates the flow of chi along the invisible meridians that flow throughout the body, linking over 100 acupoints. The basic qi gong belief is that illness results from a chi imbalance, which can be relieved through meditation, visualization, breathing and movement exercises, which restore a healthy flow to distressed parts of the body.

Qi gong exercises can be done by anyone, and are easily adapted to a wide range of physical capabilities. It has a variety of benefits, including reducing blood pressure, and enhancing oxygenation of the blood. The exercises have a beneficial effect on nerves that regulate pain response. The exercises are thought to improve the efficiency of the immune system by increasing the flow of lymphatic fluid, hastening the elimination of toxic substances and improving general health.

Some practitioners say qi gong moderates the function of the hypothalamus, pituitary and pineal glands, and the fluid surrounding the brain and spinal cord. It decreases pain, increases immunity and improves mood. Others believe it increases the amount of white blood cells, promoting the production of enzymes needed for digestion, and improving oxygen supply by increasing lung capacity. At the very least it can enhance fitness and promote relaxation.

Try it Yourself

These exercises[1] are intended to unblock the 12 meridians and improve overall health. It is recommended they each be performed three times, once or twice a day, working within your comfort level and maintaining a peaceful frame of mind. Moves should be performed very slowly.

Each position begins with what is called the "Natural Standing Form", with feet shoulder width apart, arms hanging at your sides, your back straight, spine lengthened, chin tucked and your tongue pressed lightly against the roof of your mouth.

---

[1] The exercises here were compiled using research from L. Hong and P. Perry, *Mastering Miracles, The Healing Art of Qi Gong as Taught by a Master*. See Appendix C for more information.

Exercise #1: Reach for Happiness

This movement exercises the whole body, increases blood flow and tones internal organs, and is beneficial for digestive, heart, lung, spine, back, stiff neck and eye problems.

Begin by assuming the Natural Standing Form. Keeping your armpits open throughout this exercise, imagine you're gathering a ball of energy as you lift your arms out to the side, then to the front, letting them settle palms up, fingers facing each other, just below you navel. Then raise your hands and the energy ball up to your heart, keeping your chest open. Turn your palms down and rotate your thumbs inward, interlocking your fingers. Exhale and look up as you extend your arms upward, palms up, stretching your arms as far as possible while maintaining interlocked fingers, and raising up on your toes. Inhale deeply, and as you exhale, bring your eyes and head back to a frontal position, letting your arms float down gently.

Exercise #2: The Archer

This exercise improves circulation and heart and lung function, posture and balance.

Begin in Natural Standing Form position, then step your feet farther apart and bend your knees slightly. Inhale and cross your arms in front of your heart, palms facing in, right hand closest to your body. Exhale and look at the spot where your wrists cross, concentrating on it as you curl the fingers of your right hand in a loose fist, extending your left hand, palm out. Inhale and look at your left middle finger as you push the left hand away from your body. As if you were holding a bow and arrow, pull your right hand back until it is in front of your right shoulder. Rotate your hips partially toward your left hand, and allow your legs to straighten. Focus on opening your chest and your mind. Exhale and return to crossed-hands position. Repeat with your opposite hands.

Exercise #3: Between Heaven and Earth

This exercise uplifts the stomach, spleen, liver and gallbladder, and aids digestion.

Begin in Natural Standing Form. Bring your arms out to the sides, then to the front, then just below your navel. Inhale and bring your hands in front of your solar plexus (at the top of your stomach), exhale and bring your right palm overhead, and your left down toward the floor, your eyes following your right hand. Rise up on your toes if possible. Inhale and bring your palms down to your lower ribs, fingers facing down. Exhale and slide your hands down the length of your body as far as they will go to direct bad energy out through your legs and feet. Return to starting position and switch hands.

Exercise # 4: Look Back and Let Go

This exercise brings relief from stress and related disorders, and stimulates circulation.

Begin in Natural Standing Form. Step your feet wider than shoulder width and bend your knees slightly. Inhale and bring your hands about six inches from the side of your waist, stretching thumbs out and down, palms down. Exhale and bend your knees, with your weight evenly distributed over both feet, bringing your energy just below your navel. Inhale and rotate your upper body as far left as possible, turning your head to look over your left shoulder, keeping your shoulders loose. Exhale and come back to centre. Switch sides.

Exercise # 5: Twist and Release

This exercise is beneficial for the whole body; it relieves tension and increases breathing capacity.

Begin in Natural Standing Form. Step feet wider than shoulder width apart, weight evenly distributed, and bend your knees slightly. Rest your hands on your thighs and stretch your fingers and thumbs apart, thumbs pointing back. If possible bend your knees so that your hands are close to your knees. Bring your energy to the soles of your feet, and ensure your hips and wrists are loose. Inhale and rotate your torso to the left, leading with your left shoulder, and look left. Then look over your right shoulder to your right foot. Make each movement slowly and smoothly.

Exhale, bend your right knee and return to starting position, repeating on the other side.

Exercise #6: Bending for Health

This exercise stimulates the kidneys, adrenal glands, and lower abdomen. People with serious illnesses, particularly heart disease or high blood pressure, are cautioned to do this exercise gently and not to bend too far backward or forward.

Begin in Natural Standing Form, then step your feet slightly wider than shoulder width. Inhale and bring your hands to the sides, then to the front, bringing them close to the abdomen across from the kidneys, palms facing down. Exhale and place your palms on your mid-back, thumbs front, fingers pointing back, keeping your legs straight and knees loose. Inhale, lengthen your spine and lean back as far as is comfortable, trying to bend your entire spine. Exhale and bend forward as far as possible, letting your head hang, relaxing your waist and back muscles. Inhale and straighten. Return your hands to your kidneys, lengthen your spine and look up, bending backward as far as you are comfortably able. Exhale and straighten, bringing your hands up overhead, then bend forward, effortlessly bringing your hands down, holding your knees, lower legs or toes.

Exercise # 7: Energy Punch

This exercise increases vitality, stimulates the central nervous system, lungs, skeletal and muscular systems, and promotes good blood circulation.

Begin in Natural Standing Form, then step your feet slightly wider than shoulder width apart, and bend your knees slightly. Inhale and bring your fists out to your sides then in front, in line with your shoulders. Exhale and relax your fists, bringing palms to the sides of your waist. Mentally bring your energy down just below your navel. Inhale and punch an imagined opponent slowly and forcefully, rotating your wrist so your knuckles are on top when your arm is fully extended. Exhale, return your fist to the original position, switch arms and repeat.

Exercise # 8: Energy Jump

This exercise stimulates the nervous system, skeletal system and blood circulation, and balances internal organs. Do not do this exercise if you have back problems.

Begin in Natural Standing Form, then step your left foot in so your feet are fist-width apart. Standing with your hands at your sides and your back straight, bring your arms out to gather energy then bring them back to your sides. Inhale and rise up on your toes, keeping your body relaxed, then exhale and drop back down on your heels. Do a few repetitions, then rise up on your toes and bounce up and down eight times without touching your heels to the ground. Do not repeat this bouncing portion of the exercise. Bring both hands to your lower abdomen and breathe naturally, bringing energy just below your navel. Women should place their right hand on their abdomen and cover it with their left, while men should place their left hand on their abdomen and cover it with their right.

After all eight exercises have been completed, revert back to the Natural Standing Form and breathe deeply. Imagine being fully energized, then rub your hands together and massage your face and head lightly.

Chapter Twenty Three

Treat Your Sole Mates Right with Reflexology

*If you build castles in the air, your work need
not be lost; that is where they should be. Now put
the foundations under them.*
— Thoreau

Over the course of a lifetime you can expect to walk 160,000 kilometres, the equivalent of circling the earth four times. That's a lot of pounding on the 7,000 nerve endings, 26 bones, 107 ligaments and 19 muscles found in our feet! And many fashionable shoe styles, cute though they may be, compound the impact to the detriment of our "sole mates". Fortunately there is a therapy to address this: reflexology.

Reflexology is much more than a relaxing foot massage. It's a safe, natural healing treatment that strengthens the body's healing abilities by de-stressing and relaxing it. This therapy is easily learned, and is beneficial to all ages.

History

Evidence suggests that reflexology may have been used as early as 2330 BC. Modern reflexology evolved from Zone Therapy, which surfaced in the early 20th century. Zone Therapy divides the body into 10 equal longitudinal zones running the length of the entire body, with the left thumb falling in the same zone as the left big toe, and the right thumb falling in the same zone as the right big toe. In the 1930s physiotherapist Eunice Ingham took Zone Therapy a step further, developing it into reflexology as we know it today. In addition to the 10 longitudinal zones, she added the shoulder line, diaphragm line, waist line and pelvic line lateral zones to help represent the image of the body on the feet.

What it Is

Reflexology is based on the theory that the reflexes located on the palms of the hands or the soles of the feet correspond to specific parts of the body. Stimulating specific foot reflexes reduces tension and relaxes the corresponding body part, and increases circulation, which helps promote natural functions.

What it Does

Your feet are like a microcosm of your body, with the right foot corresponding to the right side of your body, the left foot corresponding to the left side, and the toes corresponding to the head. The ball of each foot, and the same area on top of the foot, represent the corresponding side of your chest. This area contains all the chest reflexes (lungs, heart, thymus gland, breast, and shoulders). Your instep contains reflexes for all of your abdominal organs. Your heel, from the sole of your foot to the top of your ankle, contains reflexes for your pelvic area. Reflexes for your limbs are found on the outer edge of each foot.

Reflexology techniques stimulate nerve endings, increasing the flow of energy and promoting balance, restoring your body's natural state of health. By applying pressure to certain areas of your feet, a reflexologist can stimulate underactive areas or calm overactive ones.

Reflexology not only rejuvenates the body, it's a natural painkiller that can effectively treat stress-related disorders such as lower back pain, headaches and high blood pressure. It is also effective for emotional issues such as depression, sexual dysfunction and eating disorders.

A Typical Session

Each reflexology treatment and effect is unique, as each is tailored to meet individual needs. Treatments typically range from 30 to 60 minutes in duration, but the stress-relieving benefits can be experienced within minutes. During your first visit the therapist will ask you for your medical background and will explain the reflexology procedure. Then you'll be invited to relax in a reclining chair or on a treatment table while your shoes and socks are removed to allow the therapist to examine and cleanse your feet before beginning the treatment.

The therapist will apply a comfortable pressure to strategic points on your foot, asking how the pressure feels to you and adjusting it accordingly, asking you to speak up if it ever becomes painful. Though the techniques are designed to stimulate relaxation, you may feel pressure or slight discomfort in particular spots, indicating that there is congestion in the corresponding area of your body. Tension and stress can cause calcium and uric acid buildups in the feet, which put pressure on nerves and muscles, creating these tender areas. With repeated reflexology treatments these blockages will be released and any pain associated with them will disappear.

Your treatment will likely conclude with the therapist rubbing aromatherapy oil or lotion on your feet, leaving your entire body feeling relaxed and rejuvenated as your body's healing mechanisms are stimulated.

You may find you're feeling more emotional than usual as you adjust to the new flow of energy within you. As previously closed energy pathways are opened, it is natural for feelings to come up. Acknowledging these emotions will allow them to be processed and released from your body more easily. It's also recommended that you drink lots of water after a treatment, to aid the toxin elimination process.

Reflexology is beneficial during times of high stress, and can be incorporated into your regular health regime. The goal of this therapy is to unblock any congested areas and to balance the body's energies. For chronic conditions, one professional treatment a week is recommended. One treatment a month is all that is required for those in good general health. The results will last as long as the energy flow remains undisturbed.

Try it Yourself

Practising reflexology daily on your own feet can extend the benefits of these regular professional treatments, and is also a quick way to treat headaches (by rubbing your big toes), clear sinuses (by pinching the tips of the toes), even treat a hangover (by pressing the liver, kidneys, stomach and solar plexus areas).

Since every reflex area is related to a specific chakra, it's also possible to balance your chakras through reflexology. Stimulate your whole foot while visualizing the colours of the chakras as they progress from red at the base of your spine to white or gold at the top of your head.

Some benefits of reflexology include stress relief, muscle relaxation, and improved blood circulation. It also helps detoxify and cleanse your body of waste and toxins. It balances your body systems, which is essential for good health. This therapy is not recommended in the case of injuries to the feet, thrombosis, diabetes, systematic diseases, or pregnancy.

Chapter Twenty Four

Is Shiatsu for You?

Happiness is a butterfly which, when
pursued, is always beyond your grasp, but which if
you sit down quietly, may alight upon you.
—Nathaniel Hawthorne

Shiatsu, a Japanese word meaning "finger pressure", is a popular form of acupressure massage. But rather than focusing strictly on specific acupressure points, Shiatsu practitioners work the meridians to promote the flow of chi through the body. They do this by methodically holding, stretching and applying comfortable pressure to your body using their hands, elbows, knees and feet. Some forms of shiatsu also use visualization, deep breathing, stretching, meditation, and dietary advice.

History

Shiatsu's gentle, rhythmic pressure is designed to relax muscles, release tension, and encourage stress to fall away, leaving you feeling lighter, looser, and more fluid. It originated in China 2,000 years ago, and was later introduced in Japan where it became known as ancient oriental massage.

What it Is

Shiatsu works on several levels in subtle ways, and may incorporate other therapies such as chiropractic. The premise is that controlled pressure applied to the body through pressing, rubbing, rolling, pinching, and rotating will stimulate energy flow in the meridians, encouraging proper circulation of body fluids and promoting proper organ functioning. The therapists use their body weight, as opposed to muscular strength, and maintain a regular pattern of movement. The amount of pressure they use will vary, depending on the client. Treatments typically include a relaxation session, where comfortable pressure is applied to either side of the spine to relax the entire body prior to targeting specific areas.

What it Does

Japanese studies have shown shiatsu is beneficial in reducing blood pressure and heart rate as well as helping ease muscular pain, nerve conditions, carpal tunnel syndrome, migraines, low back pain, whiplash, high blood pressure, joint problems and sports injuries. Broken bones, sprains and bruises also recover more quickly with the aid of shiatsu.

Physical pain is considered to be a reflection of imbalance on the emotional, mental or spiritual level, as each level supports and affects the others. Shiatsu practitioners strive to locate and treat the source of the pain. As results are cumulative, you may be advised to have one treatment a week for a month, then as needed. You will probably feel very relaxed after a treatment, and you may also feel tired, temporarily experience cold symptoms, or you may feel emotional as the energy in your body begins to flow and rebalance. Your therapist will probably teach you stretches and exercises to do at home between treatments, and may also recommend a diet rich in whole grains, fruits, vegetables, nuts, beans and fish.

Try it Yourself

You can augment your shiatsu therapy with home treatments, using your own body weight to apply pressure to strategic points while stretching to stimulate meridians and redirect blocked energy to weakened areas. It's recommended that you wear loose fitting clothing made of natural fibres to promote the flow of energy, and that you perform the stretches in a clean, quiet room.

The following *Makko-Ho*[1] is a daily five-step routine designed to relieve stress and to energize you for your day. It should be performed in the morning prior to eating. Stretch only as far as you're comfortably able, remembering to breathe and relax. If you're pregnant, don't perform these stretches without your doctor's consent, and use the suggested modifications.

Shiatsu Stretch #1: Bend Forward, Arms Behind Back

Begin in a standing position. Inhale and place your hands behind your back, interlocking your thumbs. Exhale and gently allow your body to hang forward from the waist, letting your arms and thumbs raise behind you. Exhale and hold this position, then inhale and straighten. Repeat this stretch three to five times.

Shiatsu Stretch #2: Sitting, Legs Tucked Under

Sit on your heels with your feet crossed, toes over toes, and your back straight. Relax and breathe. Put your arms behind you, palms flat on the floor, and lean back, keeping your buttocks touching your feet, knees together. Don't arch your back. If you can't feel a stretch down the length of your thighs, rest on your elbows. Breathe. If this stretch is too easy, sit between your legs with your buttocks touching the floor and lean all the way back. Relax and breathe. Sit up in stages, propping yourself up on your elbows, then up to your palms, and then back to a full sitting position. Avoid this stretch if you have weakness or pain in your knees.

Shiatsu Stretch #3: Sitting Position

Sit on the floor with the soles of your feet touching. Inhale deeply and relax as you press your knees to floor, gently assisting with your hands if necessary. Exhale and bend forward, bringing your head as close to the floor as possible (if pregnant, avoid this stage).

---

[1] Compiled using materials from *Practising Shiatsu* (Geddes & Grosset, New Lanark, Scotland, 1999).

Relax and hold for 15 to 30 seconds, then sit up and inhale. Repeat this stretch three to five times. Then sit on your heels, palms together at chest height, elbows out and fingers touching. Inhale then exhale, extending your arms out to the side and flexing your fingers firmly. Inhale and return your hands to the first position. Repeat this stretch three to five times.

Shiatsu Stretch #4: Bend Forward, Legs Out

Sit on the floor with your back straight and your legs stretched in front of you, feet flexed toward the ceiling. Inhale. As you exhale, allow your body weight to draw you forward. Holding the soles of your feet, knees or calves, and feeling a stretch in your upper thighs, inhale and straighten. Repeat three to five times, holding the stretch for 15 to 30 seconds, continually relaxing and breathing deeply.

Shiatsu Stretch #5: Legs to Sides, Bend Forward

Sit on the floor with your legs as far apart as possible. Inhale and extend your arms toward the floor (pregnant women should stretch without letting their torso collapse or rounding their backs). Exhale and bend forward so your head touches the floor. Hold and relax for 15 to 30 seconds, then inhale and return to the upright position. Now exhale and side bend over your left leg, stretching your right arm overhead to your left. Breathe deeply and relax for 15 to 30 seconds, then inhale and return to centre. Repeat on the right side. With your legs in the same position, exhale and turn your torso to the left. Lean across your left leg, stretch and exhale. Hold and breathe for 15 to 30 seconds, then inhale and come upright. Repeat on the right side. Repeat this stretch three times.

On a warning note, shiatsu should not be applied to varicose veins, cuts or broken bones, and is not recommended for people with heart disorders, multiple sclerosis or cancer.

Chapter Twenty Five

Therapeutic Touch

The golden opportunity you are seeking is in yourself. It is not in your environment, it is not in luck or chance, or the help of others, it is in yourself alone. – Orison Swett Marden

Therapeutic touch is a therapy designed to enhance the body's ability to heal itself by easing anxieties and inducing relaxation. No direct touch is involved in this therapy. Instead, practitioners work with their hands placed on the client's energy field, that extends four to eight inches from the body, and the energy fields of the therapist and the patient interact with each other without physical contact.

History

Throughout history, cultures and civilizations all over the world have recognized and honoured individuals who heal through the "laying on of hands". The practice of therapeutic touch, however, evolved as recently as the early 1970s. It was developed by New York University nursing professor Dolores Krieger Ph.D., R.N., and self-taught healer Dora Kunz. It has since become widely practised by healthcare professionals and lay people worldwide. It is taught in over 80 universities and hospitals, and it was incorporated into the Ontario College of Nurses' *Implementation Standards of Practice* in 1990.

What it Is

The universal life force energy believed to exist in all living entities flows freely into a healthy individual's body, circulating within it and flowing out again, generating an aura outside the body. Therapeutic touch practitioners believe that they can transfer some of their energy to you, as a client, to support your energy field.

A Typical Session

A therapeutic touch treatment begins with you lying on a treatment table in a comfortable position. Often soft lighting, burning incense and relaxing music will be used to enhance the experience. The therapist will centre himself or herself through a form of meditation. Then he or she will scan your body from head to toe by passing his or her hands a few inches over you, thumbs touching and palms facing down. This enables the therapist to assess your state of health; when you are healthy, your energy field is balanced, with energy flowing through it evenly. Physical and emotional disorders will cause imbalances in your energy field, which the practitioner will strive to detect and correct.

As the practitioner gains a sense of the imbalances in your energy field, he or she begins balancing build-ups and deficiencies by moving his or her hands down and out from the top of each uneven area, redirecting the flow of energy.

The therapist will often feel different energy sensations such as tingling, heat, cold and heaviness during treatments. These sensations help the therapist to determine the type of imbalance you're experiencing, be it loose congestion, tight congestion, localized imbalances or energy deficits. Then the therapist begins the "unruffling" process, moving his or her hands in circular sweeping patterns to balance the energy, moving excess energy to areas of low energy. Once this is completed the therapist begins modulation, the final phase of the treatment, by holding his or her hands stationary over specific parts of the body that have energy imbalances.

You can expect to emerge from the treatment feeling deeply relaxed and rejuvenated. Therapeutic touch is a complementary therapy that can be used to help alleviate a wide array of physical disease, and can be used on people of all ages, as well as on animals and plants.

Chapter Twenty Six

Lighten up with Trager Bodywork

We are not human beings having a spiritual experience. We are spiritual beings having a human experience. – Teilhard de Chardin

Trager practitioners know the value of a light touch. A soft, gentle but deeply effective touch is the hallmark of Trager bodywork, which operates on the premise that a light touch will promote healing by helping your body remember the sensations of a lighter, softer way of being. It works on every level to promote relaxation and to relieve physical and emotional pain.

History

Trager is a gentle, non-intrusive therapy that operates from the inside out, rather than outside in, as with massage. It was developed by Milton Trager M.D., who introduced the therapy to the world in 1975. In Trager's view, every positive, negative or neutral experience is recorded and stored in the body and mind, and while traumatic memories can't be erased, new memories can be provided.

Believing change must occur in the mind's holding patterns for the benefits to be lasting, Trager designed his bodywork to break up negative, inhibiting body and mind patterns and to instill positive experiences and memories.

What it Does

Trager addresses physical and non-physical aspects of our being. Therapists work in a meditative state to enable them to communicate with you on a heart-to-heart, mind-to-mind level. No oils or traditional massage techniques are used, and you may be fully or partially clothed for the treatment, which takes 60 to 90 minutes.

A Typical Session

Trager therapists begin by explaining the gentle nature of the work and asking if any areas need special attention or should not be worked, stressing that there should be no discomfort whatsoever during the procedure. Using a soft touch the therapist gently manipulates your head, neck, arms, legs, and torso. By focusing on specific areas the therapist creates movement throughout your whole body, triggering response waves in the core of your body that resonate to the surface. Each wave brings increased relaxation promoting release in the body and mind.

A Trager therapist works within your pain-free range, striving to give you a sense of how to move freely and painlessly. As he or she approaches a body part the therapist will gain a sense of the "weight" of the area, which relates to the amount of tension found there. If muscle tightness is apparent the therapist works even more lightly, as opposed to other bodywork disciplines that work muscles deeper and harder when resistance is encountered. This will leave you feeling nurtured, centered and deeply relaxed.

You will be asked to participate by communicating with the therapist throughout the treatment, relaying what you feel happening as the therapist listens for the relay of the movement. The therapist will endeavour to communicate a quality of peace, love and relaxation to your nervous system during the table work, then will teach you how to continue the process with "Mentastics", mental gymnastics. Mentastics emphasize the importance of the mind's participation in movement, using Trager principles.

Mentastics

The slight movements of Mentastics loosen old, restrictive movements and postural patterns in the body and mind, enabling you to learn new, more functional patterns. By recreating the table work experience in your own home, you'll be able to integrate Trager into your daily life.

Trager's rocking, rolling, and shaking movements are reputed to provide relief from a wide range of conditions, ranging from everyday aches and pains to serious conditions such as depression, multiple sclerosis, cerebral palsy and Parkinson's disease. It also improves sports injuries or job-related ailments like carpal tunnel syndrome. It can be used to complement a preventative maintenance health program, or for simple relaxation to bring peace and transformation into your life.

Chapter Twenty Seven

Usui Reiki:

Going with the Flow

Just for today, I will give thanks for my many blessings. Just for today I will look at the positive. Just for today I will deal with anger appropriately. Just for today I will do my work honestly. Just for today I will be kind to everyone and everything. – Mikao Usui

Imagine just lying back and relaxing while pain and stress disappear, simply by having a therapist touch you. Sound too easy? The beauty of reiki is that the process really is that simple, and that profound.

The name says it all. Reiki comes from the Japanese word *rei*, meaning universal, and *chi*, meaning the energy flowing through all living things. For reiki practitioners, accessing this "ray" is "key" to facilitating healing.

Life force flows through our bodies, through our chakras and meridians, and around us through our auras, nourishing our organs and cells. It responds to thoughts and feelings, and is disrupted whenever we have conscious or subconscious negative thoughts or feelings about ourselves. Negative thoughts and feel-

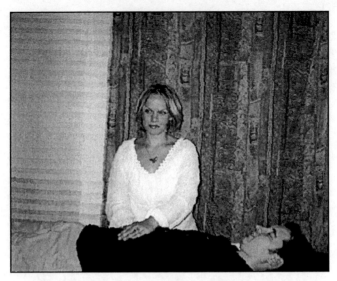

Reiki uses the flow of energy to treat emotional, physical and mental problems. Here, Reneé Leduc performs a reiki treatment on Kevin Lowery.

ings become attached to the energy field causing disruption in the flow of life force, diminishing organ and cellular function.

History

Reiki began as a Tibetan Buddhist practice some 3,000 years ago. Dr. Mikao Usui, a Japanese priest, rediscovered it in the mid-1800s and spent the rest of his life travelling throughout Japan, teaching his followers how to channel energy through themselves to promote healing in others.

What it Is

This therapy is based on the assumptions that life force energy has a source, that can be contacted and tapped. People can learn to utilize this energy easily. There are always positive results, though not always the ones you expect.

Reiki is a hands-on healing technique using a particular form of life force that can only be channelled by people who've been attuned to it. It has the ability to flow through negatively affected parts of the energy field and charge them with positive energy. This raises the vibratory level in and around the body, breaking up negative energy and clearing energy pathways, allowing life force to flow naturally.

A reiki practitioner accesses this particular form of energy, making it available for you to promote healing. It flows through the therapist's body and into you in direct proportion to your physical, mental, emotional and spiritual needs. Reiki differs from many other forms of natural healing in that it can also be conducted with the practitioner and client in different locations, and the energy will not be diminished.

During their training, reiki practitioners receive a specific initiation allowing them to tap into the universal life force. The three degrees of reiki each require a special attunement. A first degree reiki practitioner has the ability to transmit energy to any living thing by touching it. A practitioner holding a second degree is able to offer distant treatments, and to treat mental or emotional problems. At the third degree, the practitioner becomes a reiki master, and is able to teach reiki to others.

What it Does

The life force has an innate intelligence that corrects imbalances, helping the mind and body return to their own perfection. It finds its way to the areas of the body that need it most, bringing body, mind and soul into a state of harmony. It does this by balancing organs and glands, releasing repressed emotions, and promoting natural self-healing.

Physically the energy promotes balance, enabling the body to heal itself. This in turn benefits people mentally by making ordinary ups and downs more manageable, stress easier to handle, and learning easier. Reiki also encourages spiritual growth by increasing an individual's ability to meditate or pray, allowing easier access to the inner voice of guidance.

Reiki is widely regarded as a stress reducer and a preventative treatment that strengthens the immune system and relieves pain. In addition to treating physical ailments, it is reputed to help with deep emotional and mental problems such as bipolar disorder and schizophrenia. It also helps calm children with Attention Deficit Disorder (ADD). Animals and plants also benefit from reiki. It can be used to treat many conditions, from arthritis to whiplash and virtually everything in between. Reiki can also be used to balance the chakras, to harmonize the body and to dissolve energy blockages, releasing potential abilities.

A Typical Session

Your reiki treatment should be conducted in a relaxing atmosphere, which will probably include low lighting and soothing music. A professional treatment will probably begin with the reiki-ist taking a medical case history, especially if you are there for a particular problem. You'll be asked to remove shoes and restrictive clothing such as belts and ties, as well as eyeglasses, watches and other jewellery.

During treatments, which last approximately 90 minutes, you will lie on a table covered by a blanket, though treatments can also be administered while sitting or standing. After taking a moment to personally centre the energy, the therapist will lay his or her hands in strategic positions on or just above your major organs and glands, enabling the energy to flow through you to where it's needed. You may feel warm or cold sensations, tingling, a sense of lightness or heaviness, and possibly the echo of past ailments as reiki works through your system. You'll probably feel deeply relaxed during treatments; indeed, it is this state of deep relaxation that promotes the self-healing. If you don't experience any of these sensations, it only means you're not sensitive to this particular energy at this time.

Following the treatment you may want to nap while the self-healing and detoxification continues, or you might feel an increase in energy. The detoxification process may manifest itself in the form of nausea, headaches, runny nose, strong urine or loose stools. These are beneficial reactions that indicate your body is healing itself, and most people don't experience any of these symptoms to a noticeable degree. Often only three reiki treatments are required to address specific complaints; it's recommended they be taken a week apart, as the treatments have a cumulative effect. Reiki also dislodges toxins and build-ups throughout the body, which the client should flush out by drinking lots of water immediately following a treatment.

Chapter Twenty Eight

Visualization:

Be a Daydream Believer

*Visualize the thing you want. See it, feel it,
believe in it. Make your mental blueprint and
begin to build! – Robert Collier*

Want to be successful in all your ventures? First you have to become a daydream believer. Visualization is essentially using your imagination to create what you want, and is a powerful tool to help you attain goals.

History

Visualization is a simple process that has figured in East Indian Ayurvedic medicine, and used by Ancient Egyptians and North American shamans. The practice of using the mind and senses to conjure images to control pain and attain goals became popular in western medicine in the 1960s, when oncologist Carl Simonton and psychologist Stephanie Simonton had positive results treating cancer by combining conventional treatment with visualization. The uses of visualization are virtually limitless.

What it Is

Imagination is something we use every day, though we often predict difficulties, conjuring up worst-case scenarios that we unwittingly project into our reality. Fortunately, the opposite is also true. You can consciously use visualization to create what you really want from life, including health, wealth, love and inner peace.

Form follows thought, and every creation, whether it's a peanut butter sandwich or a musical masterpiece, begins in thought form. An idea creates an image of the form, then the form attracts physical energy into itself, allowing it to manifest into the physical plane. Simply put, we attract into our lives that which we expend the most mental energy on, be it negative or positive.

The process of visualization is simply using your imagination to create a life situation you truly desire, conjuring a clear image and focusing on it until it becomes a reality. The goal may be on any level: physical, mental or spiritual.

We all think constantly, day and night, but those thoughts are primarily habitual. As much as 85 per cent of our thoughts may be "recycled", dating back over a period of years. To affect change in your life, you must stop wasting energy listening to critical inner dialogue and reprogram these old patterns and internal conversations. Affirmations, thoughts you select because you desire the results they will produce, have the power to help you replace negative mind chatter with productive beneficial thought patterns, which in turn can change your life.

Affirmations should always be phrased in the most positive way, for example, "I now enjoy a harmonious relationship with my son/daughter/spouse" rather than, "I won't argue with my son/daughter/spouse any more." They should also be phrased as if they are already a reality, such as "I am a successful lawyer" as opposed to, "I will be a successful lawyer." Affirmations are particularly effective when combined with visualization; the techniques are all the more powerful because of their simplicity.

Try it Yourself

The basic principle of visualization is to relax deeply and imagine a goal exactly the way you want it to be, as if it already actually exists in reality. Focus on this goal often, giving it lots of positive energy. Early morning and late evening are good times to practise visualization, as your body is already relaxed. Deep relaxation is a vital component because it slows your busy beta brain waves to the slower, more receptive alpha level of consciousness, which is more effective in affecting changes in your life.

Begin by sitting comfortably and deep breathing, then mentally visit a place in nature where you feel most comfortable. Imagine a bright white healing light entering your body, protecting you from negative energy. Focus on your goal, be it an object or a situation. Using as many senses as you can, visualize yourself in that situation, with it unfolding just as you want it to.

Make your visualization as real as you can by adding physical dimension to it. Colour, smell, touch, texture and sound are all integral to our experience of something as real. While holding the image in your mind, say positive affirmations about it silently or aloud. Any negative thoughts that arise should be acknowledged and released, returning to your positive thoughts. Repeat this process daily. Creative visualization guru Shakti Gawain suggests following this practice by saying, "this, or something better, now manifests for me in totally satisfying and harmonious ways for the highest good of all concerned," leaving room for something even better than you imagined to occur.[1]

Do you doubt that the power of affirmations can work for you? There's an affirmation to fix that. Start by writing "my affirmations will work for me whether I believe them or not," five times a day for two weeks. This is a good procedure to follow with any affirmations, though they may not all require as much time.

The very awareness that you are the constant creator of your life gives you more control of your destiny. Affirmations and visualizations can be an effective way of achieving the life you always dreamed of.

---

[1] S. Gawain, *Creative Visualization* (New World Library, San Rafael, CA., 1995), at p. 29.

Chapter Twenty Nine

Stretch Your
Comfort Zone with Yoga

Discipline is the bridge between goals and
accomplishments. – Jim Rohn

If you're searching for a way to reduce stress, increase your fitness level and improve the quality of your life, yoga is the ideal place to begin. Unlike most exercise programs that encourage you to expend energy, yoga rewards your efforts by expanding your energy levels.

What it Is

Though it's an ancient East Indian tradition dating back 5,000 years, yoga's ideas are as vital today as they've ever been. The word *yoga* means "union and discipline". Its practice focuses on the mind/body connection. It teaches you to connect with both your body and mind on the premise that controlling your body leads to a more controlled mind. It is considered to be a path of enlightenment, with the ultimate goal of achieving a sense of oneness with the universe.

There are six paths of yoga that can lead you to *Samadhi*, self-realization: Bhakti Yoga, the devotional path, Karma Yoga, the active path, Gyana (or jnana) yoga, the philosophical path, Mantra yoga using sound, and Raja Yoga, the king of yogas. Hatha Yoga is the physical form of yoga that has been most commonly followed in the West since its surge of popularity in the 1960s, and will be the focus of this chapter.

Yoga has eight "limbs" that provide guidelines for practice as well as codes of behaviour. They include *yamas* (abstinences), *niyamas* (observances), *asanas* (postures), *pranayama* (breath control), *dharana* (concentration), *dhyana* (meditation) and *samadhi* (self-realization). These limbs promote ideas such as non-violence, truthfulness, not stealing, moderation in all things, non-possessiveness, internal and external cleanliness, contentment, observing discipline and simplicity, study of life and its meaning, and attentiveness to the divine.

What it Does

Yoga will put you more in control of your life as it tones your body and strengthens your mind through a combination of moderate exercise, deep breathing, and relaxation. In addition to its *asanas* (postures), cleansing rituals and breathing exercises are regularly practised to help manipulate body energy through breath control.

Pranayama is the yoga term for breath control. *Prana* refers to the life force or energy manifested in each of us with each breath. *Ayama* means to stretch or extend. Practising *pranayama* manipulates the life force in air for maximum physical and mental benefits, using each inhale to nourish every cell in the body with an abundance of oxygen, and each exhale to expel waste products such as stale air, leaving you feeling energized.

While it may resemble other exercise regimes on the surface (many borrow yoga moves), yoga has the potential to accomplish much more than just toning the body. There's no doubt the many *asanas* build strength and stamina through isometric strength training, but the external physical rewards are just the beginning.

Yoga helps cleanse the inner body by releasing negative energy and stimulating the lymphatic system, which filters toxins and transports nutrients to the blood. Yoga strengthens the nervous system, reduces stress, releases tension, sharpens mental faculties and increases concentration, making it an effective tool for preventing both physical and mental illness.

Beyond the many benefits, the practice of yoga also encourages meditation, putting you more in touch with yourself, and offers guidelines for living and spirituality. It transcends all cultures, religions and philosophies.

Yoga produces measurable physiological changes in the body, such as a decrease in respiratory rates and blood pressure, and altered brain wave activity that reflects relaxation. It has been shown to produce both immediate and long-term reduction of stress and anxiety. It is often recommended to relieve the pain and anxiety of chronic illness and as a complementary therapy for treating arthritis, cancer, diabetes, and many other conditions.

Try it Yourself

Yoga *asanas* can be adapted to any fitness level. Ideally, they're best learned at the hands of a competent, trained instructor who can spot and correct body alignment mistakes, but there are many books and video tapes available to get you started in your practice.

Daily yoga practice is considered to be most beneficial, with the entire body worked during each session. Any level of difficulty can be increased or decreased with modifications; participants are advised to work to their own ability and connect with what they feel as they assume the various positions. The idea is not just to work the muscles, but also to tone organs and improve internal functions, which yoga considers to be more important than muscle fitness.

Organized yoga classes typically begin with breathing exercises, move on to body postures, and finish with relaxation or meditation. Postures follow a specific order to help balance the muscle groups. Some are designed to improve posture and work the skeletal system, while others compress and relax organs and nerves. In each case the movements are performed gently, concentrating on the breath and always working within individual limitations.

Appendix A

Other Modalities to Explore

Master Alignment®: Body and Mind Alignment Through DNA Transformation™

The Master Alignment® Healing Technique identifies and removes fear-based patterns imprinted in the DNA that cause imbalances in the body and mind. Practitioners work with information and powerful energies guided by Spirit to clear the pattern from the DNA, bringing a conscious understanding and awareness of the pattern and how it affects daily life. Only one healing session is necessary as the energies allow you to clear a particular pattern, as well as other patterns that may arise in the future.

Metamorphic Technique

The Metamorphic Technique is a tool that encourages transformation from within. The therapist acts as a catalyst to release preconceived ideas and interference, allowing the client to transform in any way necessary. The therapist lightly works on spinal reflexes on the feet, hands and head, which correspond to the time before birth when characteristics are established.

Mitzvah Technique

The Mitzvah Technique is a form of bodywork that teaches how to improve body performance and how to enhance proper movement with postural corrections. It is gentle and very effective for anyone suffering from tension, stress or pain, bringing flexibility and balance to everyday movement.

Naturopathy

Naturopathic medicine provides holistic healthcare based on the belief that the body has natural healing powers, and that people's physical, mental and emotional health contribute to their overall state of health. A licensed naturopathic doctor can perform (among other things) homeopathy, herbal medicine, clinical nutrition, Chinese medicine and acupuncture, lifestyle counselling, massage, hydrotherapy, and spinal and joint manipulation.

Shamanism

Shamanism is the most ancient form of healing. It is a powerful transformational tool that uses journeying for the purpose of soul retrieval, sacred drumming, and healing. Shamans possess an understanding of the spiritual causes of disease and a respect for the laws of the universe, which enables them to help people make the changes necessary to heal the spirit.

Appendix B

Glossary

Acupoint

Pressure points located all over the body, close to the surface of the skin in small hollows, usually between bones. When these points are stimulated, pressed firmly or massaged, they have a specific effect on particular organs or body systems. There are over 360 acupoints on the body.

Aura

The word aura means "glow of light", and refers to the electromagnetic field which surrounds and permeates the body like a halo. Auras are believed to hold a record of an individual's past experiences and state of health, and change in intensity of colour, size, and shape depending on the individual's mental and emotional state.

Chakra

Chakras are energy centres aligned with the spinal chord. The human body contains seven major chakras, and 21 minor chakras. Chakras are openings for energy to flow in and out of the aura.

The seven major chakras are the crown, brow, throat, heart, solar plexus, sacral and base chakras.

Chi

Chi, also called ki or qi, refers to life energy that flows through us in channels called meridians.

Mantra

A sound used in meditation that evokes specific energies, helping stimulate the chakras as it resonates through the body. A classic example is "*ohm*", designed to make you feel at one with the universe.

Meridians

Meridians are a system of invisible channels in the body through which energy flows. They are located on both the front and back of the body. There are 12 major meridians as well a governing vessel and a directing vessel. They receive energy from organs and chakras that continually flows from one meridian to another.

Appendix C

Sources

Adamson, Eve and Budilovsky, Joan. *The Complete Idiot's Guide to Yoga.* New York, N.Y.: Alpha Books, 1998.

Bach Flower Remedies, online at <http://www.bachcentre.com>.

Brennan, Barbara Ann. *Hands of Light, A Guide to Healing Through the Human Energy Field.* New York, N.Y.: Bantam Books, 1988.

Crisp, Tony. *Dream Dictionary: An A to Z Guide to Understanding Your Unconscious Mind.* New York, N.Y.: Dell Publishing, 2002.

Dennison, Paul E., and Dennison, Gail E. *Brain Gym.* Ventura CA.: Edu-Kinesthetics, Inc., 1989.

Edwards, Victoria. *The Aromatherapy Companion.* Pownal, VT.: Storey Books, 1999.

Gawain, Shakti. *Creative Visualization.* San Rafael, CA.: New World Library, 1995.

Geddes and Grosset. *Practising Shiatsu.* New Lanark, Scotland: David Dale House, 1999.

Geddes and Grosset. *Reflexology and Complementary Therapies.* New Lanark, Scotland. David Dale House, 2002.

Gilles, Marion. *Healing from Within with Chi Nei Tsang.* New York, N.Y.: North Atlantic Books, 1999.

Holdway, Ann. *Kinesiology.* Rockport, ME.: Element, 1995.

Jensen, Bernard and Bodeen, Donald. *Visions of Health.* Garden City Park, N.J.: Avery Publishing Group, 1988.

Kelsang Gyatso, Geshe. *Meditation Handbook.* Ulverston, UK.: Tharpa Publications, 1995.

Kelsang Gyatso, Geshe. *Transform Your Life.* Ulverston, UK.: Tharpa Publications, 2001.

Kelsang Gyatso, Geshe. *Understanding the Mind.* Ulverston, UK.: Tharpa Publications, 2001.

Kluck, Michelle R. *Hands on Feet.* Philadelphia, PA.: Running Press, 2001.

Lilly, Simon. *The Complete Illustrated Guide to Crystal Healing.* Boston, MA.: Element, 2000.

Loecher, Barbara and Altshul-O'Donnell, Sara. *New Choices in Natural Healing for Women.* Emmaus, PA.: Rodale Press Inc., 1997.

McCarthy, Margot. *Natural Therapies.* London, UK.: Thorsons, 1994.

Parks, P. and C. *Reiki, The Essential Guide to the Ancient Healing Art.* London, UK.: Random House, 1998.

Peirce, Penney. *Dreams for Dummies.* Foster City, CA.: IDG Books Worldwide Inc., 2001.

Sivandanda Yoga Vedanta Centre. *Yoga Mind and Body.* Willowdale, ON.: Firefly Books, 1998.

The Upledger Institute, online at <http://www.upledger.com>.

Walls, Allen R. *Magnetic Field Therapy.* McLean, VA.: Inner Search Foundation, 1993.

Quotes for chapter openings, <http://www.insightquotes.com>.

About the Artist

Julie Champoux is the accomplished artist whose work graces the cover of this book. Julie's work is displayed at the Trenton Art Gallery, and she has converted many of her original works into a greeting card line.

Julie is a Reiki Master as well as a Trager® and Therapeutic Touch teacher and practitioner.

Alexandra Barker and Seraphine Publishing graciously thank Julie for allowing the use of her artwork in *Relief Beyond Belief.*

Julie can be reached at (613) 392-5896 or emailed at starborn333_@hotmail.com.

Complementary
Therapy Directory

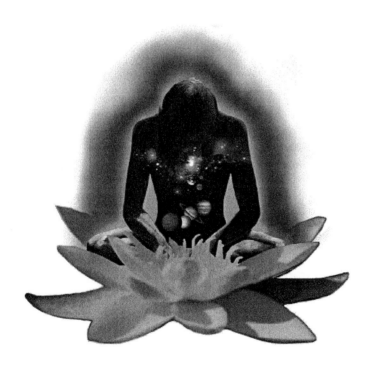

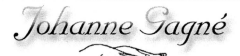
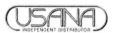
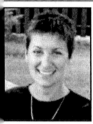
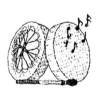
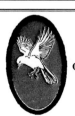

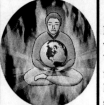

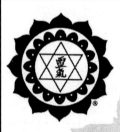
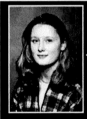
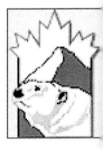

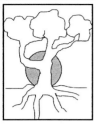
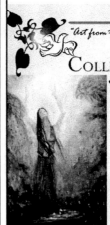
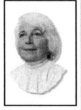

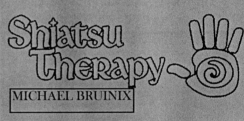

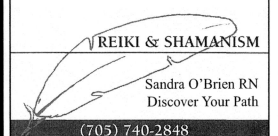

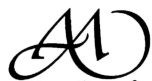
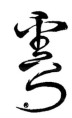

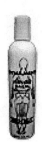
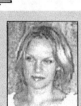

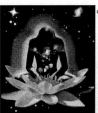

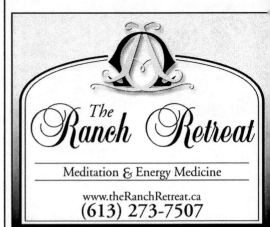
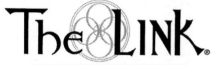